HANDBOOK of HIGH-RISK PERINATAL HOME CARE

HANDBOOK OF HIGH-RISK PERINATAL HOME CARE

HEALTH CARE RESOURCES
Rochester, New York

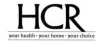

HCR
your health · your home · your choice

M Mosby

St. Louis Baltimore Boston Carlsbad Chicago Naples New York
Philadelphia Portland London Madrid Mexico City Singapore
Sydney Tokyo Toronto Wiesbaden

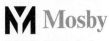

Mosby

Dedicated to Publishing Excellence

A Times Mirror
Company

Publisher Nancy L. Coon
Executive Editor N. Darlene Como
Senior Developmental Editor Laurie Sparks
Project Manager Dana Peick
Production Editor Dan Begley
Designer Amy Buxton
Manufacturing Supervisor Karen Boehme
Cover ultrasounds courtesy of Christina Buxton Martin

Printed in the United States of America
Composition by Top Graphics
Printing/binding by R.R. Donnelley & Sons, Co.

Mosby–Year Book, Inc.
11830 Westline Industrial Drive
St. Louis, Missouri 63146

ISBN 0-8151-2865-7

96   97   98   99   00   /   9   8   7   6   5   4   3   2   1

Advisory Panel

Julia Brillhart, RN, MSN
Perinatal Nurse Consultant,
Indianapolis, Indiana

June Helberg, RN, RNP, EdD
Associate Professor,
University of Rochester,
Rochester, New York

Henry M. Hess, MD, PhD
Private Practice,
Rochester, New York

M. Raymond Naassana, MD
Private Practice,
Henrietta, New York

Marie Shelanskey, MSEd, RN
Former Associate Professor,
Finger Lakes Community College,
Canandaigua, New York

Preface

This *Handbook of High-Risk Perinatal Home Care* is intended as a companion to HCR's *High-Risk Perinatal Home Care Manual*. While the *Manual* discusses such issues as the emergence of home health as a high-risk perinatal care site, the composition of the care team and the home case management model, and operational issues about quality, ethics, and risk, the *Handbook* is specifically designed for a more narrowed audience of front-line perinatal nurses in a community setting.

This *Handbook* is an easy-to-use resource that community health nurses can bring with them into the home setting as a reference aid for issues they may encounter as high-risk perinatal nurses. For a variety of specific risks, the *Handbook* includes step-by-step interventions and care plans, each divided into categories such as risk condition and definition, pathophysiology, assessments and interventions, and patient and family teaching. Tables and charts providing summary information on laboratory values, medications, maternal and fetal assessments, and electronic fetal surveillance are included in the Appendixes.

While predominantly the work of Susan Wright, RN, CHN, and specialist in perinatal home health nursing, and Peggy Edwards, MS, RN, and HCR's Director of Patient Services and Vice President for Clinical Services, this *Handbook* represents the collective wisdom and effort of our administrative support staff and the professional and paraprofessional team members who took HCR's high-risk perinatal home care program from the drawing board to the real world, caring enough about the work of front-line nurses to suggest we share our knowledge in the form of this *Handbook*.

We hope you find the *Handbook* valuable to you in your work and equally valuable to your patients in helping them attain health and well-being throughout their lives.

Louise Woerner
Chief Executive Officer
August 26, 1996

Contents

Chapter 1

Introduction

Until very recently high-risk perinatal services accounted for no more than 2% of a typical home health agency's practice. As acute health care services shifted from hospital to home, however, it was inevitable that high-risk perinatal services would do so as well.

For many reasons traditional practices are changing dramatically. As diagnostic and treatment modalities for high-risk mothers become more sophisticated and portable, home care is playing a greater role in managing complicated pregnancies. For the community health nurse of a home health agency delivering or preparing to deliver high-risk perinatal services, this handbook is offered as a template of patient assessment, interventions, home care screening, and care planning. The larger work from which this handbook is derived is Health Care Resources' (HCR's) *High-Risk Perinatal Home Care Manual,* a comprehensive text describing clinical, fiscal, legal, and quality issues involved in developing and implementing a high-risk perinatal home care program.

DEFINING THE HIGH-RISK OBSTETRIC PATIENT

A high-risk obstetric patient is defined as one who has one or more of the following:

- A current diagnosis of a pregnancy-related complication (preterm labor, preeclampsia, hyperemesis gravidarum)
- An obstetric history that places her at greater-than-average risk for the development of a pregnancy complication (multiple preterm deliveries)
- A nonobstetric medical or psychosocial history that presents a threat to maternal or fetal outcome (cardiac or renal disease, high-risk lifestyle or behavior)

Ideally every pregnant woman should be screened for her risk status in the first trimester of pregnancy by the primary care provider or case manager so that appropriate monitoring, teaching, and interventions may be instituted. The risk assessment should include a complete physical examination and an obstetric, medical, and psychosocial history; this assessment should be repeated around midpregnancy.

THE HOME CASE MANAGEMENT MODEL

The success of home-managed high-risk pregnancy is dependent on three basic elements: a motivated patient, qualified care providers, and the coordination of services. The home health care team is a multidisciplinary group in which each person serves a distinct and separate role, and the team's combined efforts and communication result in the assurance of optimal patient care and safety. This is accomplished using the nursing case management model described.

Potential team members include the following:

Team Member	Role
The patient*	Is a key player in the plan of care
	Participates in care planning and implementation
	Notifies the case manager or primary care provider when her condition or needs change
The patient's support network*	Consists of a group of informal care providers
	Carries out errands
	Provides child care
	Helps with transportation
	Prepares meals

*Denotes minimum team composition; other team members may be added as required and allowed by the payer.

Continued

Team Member	Role
Primary care provider*	Offers emotional support to the patient
	May include family, friends, neighbors, and community resources
	Refers the patient for home care
	Collaborates with the case manager in the development of the plan of care
	Orders services
	Renders primary medical care
Primary community health nurse (CHN)* or case manager*	Provides direct patient care and teaching
	Serves as the coordinator for other services
	Works in close collaboration with the primary care provider and is responsible for a safe plan of care
	Must have extensive experience in perinatal nursing
Home health aide	Provides child care, personal care, and homemaking services to assist the patient in carrying out ordered activity limitations
	Should be specifically trained in child care
Medical social worker	Evaluates psychosocial needs and makes appropriate community resource referrals to meet needs
	Assesses coping ability
	Provides counseling as needed

*Denotes minimum team composition; other team members may be added as required and allowed by the payer.

Continued

Team Member	Role
Dietician	Evaluates nutritional status
	Devises a diet plan to meet the patient's nutritional needs
	Is especially helpful for patients with hyperemesis, diabetes, and gastrointestinal disorders
Individual certified in electronic fetal surveillance (EFS)	Provides services such as non-stress testing (NST), ultrasound (US), and biophysical profile (BPP)
	May be a staff perinatal home care nurse or a consultant
Laboratory	Provides testing services to enhance clinical information
	Reports results to case manager and primary care provider
Durable medical equipment and supplies provider	Provides items such as infusion pumps, home uterine monitors, or other supplies needed to carry out the plan of care
Physical therapy providers	May evaluate and teach patients when long-term bed rest or underlying medical conditions create the potential for musculoskeletal compromise

An evaluation at the time of referral or during the first home care visit is performed to determine the individual patient's needs; the team is constructed accordingly. Team members may be added or deleted during the course of care as a reflection of changing needs or payer requirements.

ETHICAL ISSUES

Ethical dilemmas* arise from many factors, particularly from the development of new technologies that become widely used before their social and ethical impact can be considered. Recent advances in reproductive technologies, endocrinology, genetics, and neonatal, maternal, and fetal medical care have created numerous ethical dilemmas for both the recipient of care and the caregiver.

The following are examples of ethical dilemmas that can arise in perinatal practice.

- Voluntary pregnancy termination
- Selective reduction in multiple gestation
- Previable termination of pregnancy for maternal reasons
- Harvesting of fetal organs or tissues
- In vitro fertilization and decisions for the remaining fertilized ova
- Allocation of resources in pregnancies complicated by substance abuse and other antisocial behaviors
- Fetal surgery
- Use of maternal serum alpha-fetoprotein (MSAFP), amniocentesis, chorionic villus sampling (CVS) diagnosis, routine ultrasonography to make pregnancy termination decisions

---

*A dilemma is defined by *Webster's New World Dictionary,* ed 3, New York, 1991, Simon & Shuster, as (1) an argument necessitating a choice between equally unfavorable and disagreeable alternatives; (2) any situation in which one must choose between unpleasant alternatives; and (3) any serious problem.

- Maternal rights versus fetal rights
- Extraordinary medical treatment of pregnancy complications

LEGAL RISKS

Whenever the patient population can be described as "high-risk," the risks for legal difficulties increase because of the increased possibility of less-than-optimal outcomes. In addition, people are more inclined to sue over something that happens to their child than over something that happens to themselves. Anger and a need to blame are responses that occur universally during the process of grief. It is during this phase that the risk of legal action against care providers is highest. Angelini and Gibes (1987) identified the following factors contributing to perinatal lawsuits:

- Injury to or death of the infant
- Urging of family and friends
- Expensive continued care of the infant
- Anger, need to blame
- Complicated grief
- Unrealistic expectations or inadequate information for consent to care
- Expectation of profit
- Poor rapport with or mistrust of care provider(s)

DOCUMENTATION GUIDELINES

Complete, accurate, and up-to-date patient records are the key to facilitating two important issues:

- **High standard of care**—Per diem staff must have immediate access to the home care course, trends in maternal and fetal status, and remaining teaching needs so that their time may be used most efficiently and beneficially for the patient.
- **Reimbursement**—Charting the *positive effects* of rendered care on the patient's status assists in justification of visits.

The following guidelines will help to ensure that documentation is complete and accurate.

Home Care Screening

Document the patient's environment in relation to the care planned, considering such issues as whether the bed and bath will be on one floor and if the patient will have access to a phone. Record a statement of commitment to the care plan from both the patient and her support network.

Admission

Documentation of the admission visit should include the following:

- Patient's name, address, telephone number, and record number
- Name of patient's insurance company or other billing information
- Party to call in case of emergency

- Primary provider's name, address, and telephone number
- Primary, secondary, and other diagnoses
- Checklist of orders for home care and demonstration of appropriateness
- Complete record of maternal and fetal assessment
- Record of nursing, social work, and other professional interventions
- Record of patient and support network teaching done
- Detailed description of the intended care plan, including frequency of visits, reporting parameters, future interventions, and teaching
- Consent form as required by program

Future Visits

Document the assessments, interventions, and teaching accomplished. Record the evolving needs of the patient as required by status. Record the plan for the next visit, primary care appointments, and visits by other staff. Document EFS as per instructions located in Appendix 4.

Care Coordination

Record the case conferences held concerning each patient and retain this information in the patient's record. Each member of the health care team should document activities involved in coordinating care and communicate this information with other team members and the payer.

General Rules of Thumb

After the initial visit, only those areas related to the patient's diagnosis or problem list need be addressed in documentation. The exception to this is any new problem or diagnosis that arises during the home care course; either of these will require updates of the care plan and the possible addition of assessments, interventions, or team members.

In the event that a patient requires a level of care higher than that provided in the home, document the assessment leading to this decision, the notification of the primary care provider and payer source, and the mode of transportation used to bring the patient to the acute facility. Record the patient's status before, during, and after the transfer, and the name of the receiving health professional and unit to which the patient is admitted.

As with all nursing documentation, record only objective information (things that are observable and measurable) in the patient record and avoid judgmental terminology. Include any subjective information given by the patient or support network during interviewing or offered during visits.

Chapter 2

Management of Pregnancy Complications at Home

HYPEREMESIS GRAVIDARUM

Definition

Hyperemesis gravidarum may be defined as severe nausea and vomiting associated with weight loss, ketonuria, electrolyte imbalance, and dehydration (Cunningham, 1993). It typically originates in the first trimester and is resolved by the twenty-eighth week, though it may persist throughout the pregnancy (Creasy, 1984; Connon, 1995).

Incidence

Pernicious nausea and vomiting occur in 0.3% to 1.0% of pregnancies (Connon, 1995). Hyperemesis is most prevalent in Caucasian women and is most commonly seen in first pregnancies (Connon, 1995).

Etiology

There is no particular known cause of hyperemesis in pregnancy, though theories have been advanced pointing to the culpability of certain hormone elevations, including estrogen, human chorionic gonadotropin (HCG), and thyroxine (Soules et al, 1980; Bouillon et al, 1982; Depue et al, 1987). There are several literature references to a possible psychogenic etiology:

    Nulliparity
    Obesity
    Caucasian descent
    Multifetal pregnancy

> Decreased gastric motility
> Molar pregnancy
> Psychologic factors
> *(Creasy, 1984; Williams, 1991; Cunningham, 1993; Connon, 1995.)*

Associated Risks

MATERNAL	FETAL AND NEONATAL
Dehydration	Intrauterine growth retardation (IUGR)
Sodium depletion	
Weight loss	Spontaneous abortion
Vitamin B deficiency	
Wernicke's encephalopathy	
Liver and renal damage	

 Pathophysiology

PARAMETER	NORMAL PHYSIOLOGIC CHANGE	PATHOPHYSIOLOGIC CHANGE
Hematocrit	33%-44%	Hemoconcentration
Hemoglobin	12%-15%	
Temperature (T)	97.5° F-99° F	May be febrile
Skin turgor	Optimal	May be poor
Heart rate	Increase of 10-15 beats per minute (BPM) above prepregnancy rate	Tachycardia (>20 BPM above prepregnancy rate)
Serum sodium	130-140 mg/dl	<130 mg/dl
Weight		
	Steady gain	Poor gain or loss, possibly with ketonuria

Continued

Parameter	Normal Physiologic Change	Pathophysiologic Change
B-complex vitamins	Within normal limits	Deficiency, may lead to pyelonephritis or Wernicke's encephalopathy
Liver function	Bile concentration	Jaundice
Fetal growth	Appropriate for gestational age	May be growth-retarded

 Signs & Symptoms

Early symptomatology, beginning at about 6 weeks' gestation, includes near constant nausea and pernicious vomiting. Weight loss may be present, generally at least 5 lb from baseline, and the total loss may exceed 30 lb. Signs of dehydration, such as poor skin turgor, an increase in urine concentration or decreased output, weight loss, and electrolyte depletion, may be present. Progressive symptoms may include signs of starvation, such as ketonuria, skeletal muscle wasting, significant weight loss (more than 20 lb), and fetal growth retardation. In severe cases there may be liver damage (evidenced by jaundice) or renal sequelae, such as pyelonephritis.

 Screening for Appropriateness of Home Care

Initial screening may be done in the hospital, physician's office, or at home, depending upon the severity of the illness. If the patient has been treated in the hospital on an outpatient basis with intravenous (IV) fluid bolus, a same-day home care admission may be requested. Criteria for safe care in the home include the following:

> Commitment to the plan of care from the patient and support network
>
> Support persons to allow patient to get needed rest (child care, run errands)
>
> Clean environment and storage for IV supplies for hydration and nutrition
>
> Capacity of patient and primary caregiver to learn use of equipment prn

Recommended medical safety criteria include the following:

> No evidence of impending spontaneous abortion (low abdominal cramping, vaginal bleeding)
>
> Not severely dehydrated
>
> Stable hepatic and renal function

 Home Management

Orders for home care may include the following:

> Specific limited oral (PO) diet in place of or following a nonoral (NPO) diet
>
> Antiemetic medication
>
> IV fluid infusion, possibly with multivitamins
>
> Continuous enteral infusion
>
> Total parenteral nutrition
>
> Skilled nursing visits

Skilled nursing assessment and interventions should include the following:

ASSESSMENT	INTERVENTION
Hydration	Maintain IV infusion or enteral infusion as ordered.
Skin turgor	
Dipstick urinalysis (U/A) for specific gravity	Administer PO fluids as they can be tolerated.
Venipuncture for electrolyte panel as ordered	Notify physician of signs and symptoms of worsening dehydration.
Nutrition	Maintain total parenteral nutrition (TPN) as ordered.
Daily weights	Advance PO diet as it can be tolerated.
Dipstick U/A for ketones	Report ketonuria or weight loss >5 lbs/wk.
Nausea and vomiting	Administer antiemetic as ordered.
	If on enteral infusion, stop infusion × 1 hr, restart at lowest rate, and increase as ordered.
	Limit activity and provide minimal stimulation.
	Notify provider of protracted vomiting.
Fetus	Notify provider of fetal heart rate (FHR) <110 BPM or >160 BPM.
FHR activity	Notify provider for decreased fetal movement.
Fetal growth (measure fundal height)	Notify provider for fundal height >3 cm below gestational age in weeks.
Pregnancy integrity	Notify provider of uterine contractions, vaginal bleeding, or signs and symptoms of infection.

Continued

Assessment	Intervention
Safety	Change nasogastric (NG) tube weekly, bag and tubing daily.
Assess enteral infusion set	Rotate peripheral IV sites q 3 days.
Assess IV site	Change long-life catheter dressing 3 times/wk.
	Report signs and symptoms of site infection.
Coping	Explain pathophysiology and therapy.
	Encourage venting of feelings.
	Refer to support groups.
	Provide appropriate printed literature.

Patient Health Teaching

Pertinent health teaching should include instruction on the following:

> Using and caring for NG tube, enteral feeding pump, and related supplies
>
> Using and caring for IV site, tubing, solutions, and supplies
>
> Troubleshooting infusion equipment
>
> Reintroducing PO diet
>
> Signs and symptoms to report
>
>> Protracted vomiting
>>
>> Significant dehydration or malnutrition
>>
>> Hepatic or renal symptoms
>>
>> Decreased fetal movement
>>
>> Uterine contractions
>>
>> Abnormal vaginal discharge

Equipment and supply list includes the following:

For enteral infusion:
- Enteral infusion pump and instruction book
- IV pole
- Bag and tubing sets
- 8 French NG tubes
- 10-cc syringes with catheter tips
- Clear adhesive tape
- Feeding solution

For IV infusion:
- IV pole
- IV solution
- Tubing sets
- Pump or flow regulators
- Peripheral IV catheters or long-life catheters
- Normal sterile saline flush
- 3-cc syringes
- Sharps container if not using needleless system
- IV start kits
- Clear adhesive dressings
- Paper tape

The authors recommend long-life catheters for probable prolonged or chronic intermittent IV therapy.

CERVICAL INCOMPETENCE

Definition

Cervical incompetence is defined as painless cervical dilation occurring in midtrimester (Cunningham, 1993). Diagnosis may be made following two or more spontaneous midtrimester pregnancy losses and after differential diagnoses have been ruled out (Niebyl, 1994).

Incidence

Cervical incompetence occurs in 0.1% to 1.0% of all pregnancies and is the cause of up to 25% of all spontaneous abortions occurring in midtrimester (Niebyl, 1994).

Etiology

The causes of cervical incompetence include the following congenital and acquired factors:

Uterine anomalies, such as bicornate uterus

Structural abnormalities of the cervix and lower uterine segment, often found in women exposed to diethylstilbestrol (DES) in utero

Cervical trauma, including lacerations caused by precipitous or operative delivery, previous artificial dilation for curettage, cervical biopsy, or multiple induced abortions

Increased levels of relaxin

(Haning et al, 1985; Ansari et al, 1987; Parisi, 1989; Niebyl, 1994.)

Associated Risks

MATERNAL	FETAL AND NEONATAL
Midtrimester pregnancy loss	Prematurity
Preterm labor or premature delivery	Death
Preterm premature rupture of membranes	
Chorioamnioitis	
Cesarean section	
Uterine rupture	

(Ansari, 1987; Parisi, 1989; Roberts, 1990; Robichaux, 1990; Cunningham, 1993.)

 Pathophysiology

PARAMETER	NORMAL PHYSIOLOGIC CHANGE	PATHOPHYSIOLOGIC CHANGE
Obstetric history	<2 spontaneous 2nd trimester abortions	≥2 spontaneous 2nd trimester abortions
Uterocervical structure	Normal	May be anomalous or damaged
Cervix, before 37th wk	Long, thick, closed	Dilated and effaced to some degree
Membranes	Intact	May be ruptured
Uterine fundus	Soft	May be contractile

 Signs & Symptoms

As previously stated the dilation of the cervix in women with cervical incompetence occurs painlessly. Women with this condition are usually unaware of uterine contractions, though recent literature suggests that cervical incompetence may actually be early preterm labor that the patient cannot feel. Some women may have subtle warning signs for several days including perineal or lower abdominal pressure, urinary frequency, and increased (possibly bloody) vaginal discharge (Niebyl, 1994).

Screening for Appropriateness of Home Care

As always, careful assessment to ensure that the patient and plan are appropriate for home management is one of the keys to safe and effective care. General criteria include the following considerations:

> General cleanliness of the home
>
> Level of commitment to and participation in the plan of care on the part of patient and support network
>
> Degree to which environment is suited to physical activity limitations

Suggested medical criteria include the following:

> Stable cervical status
>
> No evidence of preterm labor OR uterine activity successfully suppressed
>
> No evidence of fetal compromise

Home Management

The patient with cervical incompetence may have undergone a procedure such as transvaginal cervical cerclage or transabdominal cervicoisthmus cerclage. She may be taking oral or parenteral tocolytic therapy and may be using a home uterine monitor because of the risk of preterm labor. Orders may include the following:

Skilled nursing visits for assessment, interventions, and pertinent teaching

Tocolytic therapy

Laxative or stool softener

Bed rest or limited physical activity

Home uterine monitoring

Skilled nursing assessments, interventions, and teaching should include the following:

ASSESSMENT	INTERVENTION
Pregnancy integrity Rupture of membranes Contractility Perineal pressure	Notify provider of rupture of membranes, increased uterine activity, vaginal bleeding, or perineal pressure.
	Monitor uterus at home as ordered.
	Administer tocolytics as ordered.
Safety Potential for infection	Notify provider of purulent vaginal discharge, maternal T >101° F, or fetal tachycardia.
Fetus	Notify provider of decreased fetal movement or fundal height measurement 3 cm less than gestational age in weeks.
Coping	Explain pathophysiology of condition.
	Explain plan of care.
	Allow venting of fears and feelings.
	Link with support group.
	Provide printed literature regarding prematurity and a video tour of neonatal intensive care unit (NICU).

Patient Health Teaching

Pertinent health teaching should foster awareness of the following:

Ordered activity (bed rest)

Danger of Valsalva maneuver

Dietary adjustments to minimize constipation or straining at stool (fruit juices, fiber)

Signs and symptoms to report

Regular contractions

Perineal pressure

Change in vaginal discharge

Low back pain or pressure

Change in availability of support network or environment

Signs for which immediate transfer to hospital is indicated

Strong contractions less than 5 minutes apart

Rupture of membranes

Severe perineal pressure

Urge to push

Therapeutic use and side effects of medications as necessary

Use of home monitoring equipment as necessary

HYPERTENSIVE DISORDERS IN PREGNANCY

Definition

Hypertension in pregnancy is categorized into two main types:

Chronic—hypertensive state predates the pregnancy

Gestational—hypertensive state occurs during the pregnancy, usually after 20 weeks' gestation

These conditions may be further classified as follows:

Hypertension	Systolic blood pressure (SBP) >140 mm Hg
	Diastolic blood pressure (DBP) >90 mm Hg
Severe hypertension	SBP >160 mm Hg or DBP >110 mm Hg on two occasions at least 6 hr apart
Gestational hypertension	Hypertension occurring after the 20th wk of gestation or during the early postpartum period
Preeclampsia	Hypertension
	Proteinuria of 2+ by dipstick or >300 mg in 24 hr on two occasions at least 4 hr apart with UTI ruled out

Continued

Severe preeclampsia	Severe hypertension
	PLUS ANY OR ALL OF THESE:
	Proteinuria of ≥3+ by dipstick or >5 g in 24 hr
	Urine output of <400 ml/24 hr or consistent output of <30 ml/hr
	Severe headache or visual disturbances
	Epigastric pain
	Pulmonary edema
	Platelet count <100,000/ml
Hemolysis, elevated liver enzymes, and low platelet count (HELLP) syndrome	Hemolysis
	Elevated liver enzymes (aspartate amino-transferase) >70 international units per liter
	Low platelet count (<100,000/ml)
Eclampsia	Gestational hypertension with seizure or coma

(ACOG Tech. Bulletin #91; Working Group, 1990; Sibai, 1991; Cunningham and Gant, 1993.)

Incidence

Hypertension is present in nearly 10% of all pregnancies (Working Group, 1990), with a higher incidence occurring among nulliparous and multifetal pregnancies and in women who have had preeclampsia in a previous pregnancy (Sibai, 1991).

Etiology

The exact cause of gestational hypertension remains unknown (Sibai, 1991; Roberts, 1994). However, the following risk factors for the disease have been identified:

Less than 19 or greater than 40 years of age
Nullipara
Chronic hypertension
Hypertension in a previous pregnancy other than the first
Familial history of gestational hypertension, particularly eclampsia
Multifetal pregnancy
Diabetes
Hydrops fetalis
Hydatidiform mole
(Working Group, 1990; Cunningham and Gant, 1993.)

Black women are at no greater risk for the development of preeclampsia between ages 20 and 35 (Saftlas et al, 1990). However, the incidence of preeclampsia rises significantly after age 35 in black women because the prevalence of chronic hypertension in black women is two to three times that of white women and because chronic hypertension carries a 70% incidence of superimposed preeclampsia (Working Group, 1990).

Associated Risks

MATERNAL	FETAL AND NEONATAL
Placental abruption	IUGR
Disseminated intravascular coagulopathy	Preterm birth
Cerebral hemorrhage	Demise
Acute renal failure	
Acute heart failure	
Death	

(Rochat et al, 1988; Cunningham and Gant, 1993.)

Preeclampsia and eclampsia are the second leading causes of maternal mortality (Saftlas et al,
1990), accountable for 12% of maternal deaths in
the United States (Rochat et al, 1988).

 Pathophysiology

Although it is categorized as a hypertensive disorder, preeclampsia is a "complex clinical syndrome potentially involving all organ systems"
(Friedman et al, 1991). The subjective symptomatology of both severe preeclampsia and HELLP
syndrome is manifestations of vasospasm, called
the "single event common to each of the affected
organ systems" (Gilstrap and Gant, 1990). Current
literature speculates that pregnancy-induced hypertension may arise from a failure of trophoblas-
tic tissue migration, increased sensitivity to vaso-
pressors, decreased plasma volume, and increased
resistance of the renal tubules (Walsh, 1990; Friedman, 1991). The following table outlines the specific changes associated with the disease:

PARAMETER	NORMAL PHYSIOLOGIC CHANGE	PATHOPHYSIOLOGIC CHANGE
Blood volume	50% increase	Lesser increase
Plasma volume	Increased	Small or no increase
Hematocrit	Physiologic anemia	Hemoconcentration
Cardiac output	40%-50% increase	Variable
Blood pressure (BP)	Decline, then return to prepregnancy level	Hypertension

Continued

PARAMETER	NORMAL PHYSIOLOGIC CHANGE	PATHOPHYSIOLOGIC CHANGE
Peripheral vascular resistance	Decline	Increased
		Increased vascular reactivity; vasospasm
Renal function	Increased perfusion	Decreased
Renal plasma flow	75% increase	Decreased
Glomerular filtration rate (GFR) by 2nd trimester	50% increase	Decreased
	Decreased urea nitrogen	Increased urea nitrogen
	Creatinine clearance	Increased creatinine (Decreased clearance)
	Decreased uric acid	Increased uric acid
Renin-angiotensin-aldosterone system	Markedly increased, appropriately to posture and salt intake	Renin concentration and activity suppressed; loss of vasodilators to angiotensin II
Coagulation system	Increased	Initially normal
Fibrinogen		Increased in severe preeclampsia
Factors VII, VIII, IX, X	All increased	Consumption of Factor VII
Fibrinolytic activity	Decreased	Increased
Platelet count	Normal or slightly increased	Decreased
Bleeding time	Normal	Prolonged

(Roberts, 1994.)

Signs & Symptoms

Early evidence of gestational hypertensive disease includes the following signs:

> BP elevation greater than 140/80 mm Hg
> Edema of lower extremities after 8 hours lying down
> Weight gain of greater than 4 lb in 1 week

Proteinuria may not be present in the early stages of the disease process (Sibai, 1991; Burrow and Ferris, 1995).

 Screening for Appropriateness of Home Care

The screening process, necessary to ensure a safe plan of care at home, may be performed by a discharge planner (if the patient is referred by the hospital) or by the CHN at the first home visit (if the patient is referred by the physician's office). The following criteria should be met:

- Patient meets medical criteria for hypertension, gestational hypertension, or mild preeclampsia.
- Patient and support network are motivated to participate in plan of care.
- Environment satisfies patient's need for minimal stress (atmosphere is calm) and convenience (bedroom, bath, and telephone on same floor).

Conversely, the following criteria may indicate that a particular patient is NOT appropriate for home care:

- Patient's medical condition is regarded as severe hypertension or severe preeclampsia.
- Patient or support network are unwilling or unable to fully participate in the plan of care.
- Environment is unsuited to patient's needs because of high levels of chaos and stress or physical inconveniences (no phone handy).

 Home Management

Orders for home care interventions vary among primary care providers but may include the following:

Bed rest with bathroom privileges

Regular or modified diet

Antihypertensive medication or sedative

Skilled nursing assessment of maternal and fetal well-being

Daily fetal movement counting

Daily weight measurements

EFS: US, NST, or BPP

Pertinent health teaching provided to patient and family and support network

Urine output measurements

Urine protein measurements

Skilled nursing assessments and interventions at each visit should include the following:

| | MATERNAL | |
ASSESSMENT	INTERVENTION
Vital signs	Report SBP >140 mm Hg or DBP >80 mm Hg at rest.
	Transfer to hospital for SBP >160 mm Hg or DBP >110 mm Hg at rest.
Urine dipstick for protein	Report 2+ or greater.
Deep tendon reflexes	Report 3+ or greater.
Pulmonary assessment	Transfer to hospital for adventitious lung sounds or respiratory distress.
Urine output	Report output <800 ml/24 hr.
	Transfer to hospital for output <400 ml/24 hr.
Weight	Report >2 lb gain/day or 4 lb/wk.
Subjective	Transfer to hospital for epigastric pain, visual disturbances, or severe headache.

| | FETAL |
ASSESSMENT	INTERVENTION
FHR	Report FHR >160 BPM or <110 BPM.
	Transfer to hospital if FHR cannot be auscultated.
Fundal height	Report variation of 2 cm or more from gestational age in weeks or growth of <1 cm/wk up to 38 wk.
Fetal movement	Transfer to hospital for patient report of decreased fetal movement in last 24 hr or no fetal movement in last 4 hr.
NST*	Report reassuring strip.
	Transfer to hospital for nonreassuring strip.
US*	Report results.
BPP*	Report results.

*See Appendix 4.

Patient Health Teaching

The patient and her support network should be instructed on the plan of care, the importance of cooperating with it, and the signs and symptoms or changes that should be reported to the CHN or primary care provider.

Pertinent health teaching should include instruction in the following areas:

Bed rest in left-lateral position

Maintaining a quiet, calming environment (low lighting, minimal noise, few visitors, appropriate child care)

Therapeutic use and side effects of medications

Fetal movement counting

Obtaining and documenting urine output and daily weight

Signs and symptoms to report

Weight gain of 2 lb in 1 day

Increased edema, particularly of hands or face

Urine output of less than 800 ml in 24 hours

Decreased fetal movement in last 24 hours

Change in safety of plan, including loss of appropriate environment

Decreased support network availability

Signs and symptoms for which immediate transfer to hospital is indicated

Epigastric or right-sided chest pain

Visual disturbance

Severe headache

Urine output of less than 400 ml in 24 hours

No fetal movement in 4 hours

In the early phase of the home care course, visits should be frequent (daily if possible) to establish baseline assessments, ensure an adequate environment and support network, and accomplish teaching necessary to ensure patient safety in the time between visits.

PLACENTAL ABNORMALITIES

Two types of placental abnormality that may be managed with home care include placental abruption (abruptio placentae) and placenta previa. Though these conditions are very different, the similarities between them concerning maternal and fetal risks, management objectives, and interventions are such that the conditions are presented together.

Definitions

Placental abruption, or abruptio placentae, is a premature separation of the placenta from the uterine wall after 20 weeks' gestation (Cunningham et al, 1993). An abruption may be concealed (occurring inside the margins, with no vaginal bleeding seen) or apparent or marginal (occurring at or near the margins with vaginal bleeding present) (Gilbert and Harmon, 1993).

Placenta previa describes a low-lying placenta that is attached very near the cervical os (marginal previa), partially covering it (partial previa), or totally covering it (complete previa) (Cunningham et al, 1993).

Incidence

Placental abruption occurs in 0.8% to 1.8% of all pregnancies and the recurrence risk is 5% to 15% (Pritchard, 1970; Fox, 1978; Lowe and Cunningham, 1990).

Placenta previa occurs in 0.5% of all pregnancies (Lavery, 1990).

Etiology

The precise cause of placental abruption is unknown. Several factors that increase the risk of abruption have been identified:

Hypertension

Short umbilical cord

Maternal trauma

Previous abruption

Sudden uterine decompression

Premature rupture of membranes

Folic acid deficiency

Uterine anomaly

Cigarette smoking

Cocaine use

(Pritchard et al, 1970; Crosby and Costila, 1971; Naeye et al, 1977; Lehtoverta and Forss, 1978; Karegaard and Gennser, 1968; Vintzileos et al, 1987; Janke, 1990; Hoskins et al, 1991; Floyd et al, 1991.)

The cause of placenta previa, like the cause of abruption, is unknown. The following list contains known risk factors for implantation of the placenta in the lower, rather than fundal, segments of the uterus:

Multiparity

Endometrial scarring from multiple therapeutic abortions or uterine surgeries

Inadequate endometrial blood supply, as from chronic disease, drug use, or cigarette smoking

Male fetus

(Cotton et al, 1980; Fraser and Watson, 1989; Green, 1989; Williams et al, 1991.)

Associated Risks

ABRUPTION	
MATERNAL	**FETAL AND NEONATAL**
Hemorrhagic shock	Hypoxia
Disseminated intravascular coagulopathy (DIC)	Prematurity
Renal failure	IUGR
Postpartum hemorrhage	Death
Rhodium (Rh) sensitization	
Pituitary necrosis	
Anemia	
Endometritis	
Death	

(Hurd et al, 1983; Pritchard, 1985; Sholl, 1987; Lowe and Cunningham, 1990; Voigt et al, 1990; Konje et al, 1994.)

PREVIA	
MATERNAL	**FETAL AND NEONATAL**
Hemorrhage or hypovolemic shock	Prematurity
Placenta accreta/increta/percreta	Small for gestational age
Premature rupture of membranes	Malpresentation
Postpartum hemorrhage	Congenital anomalies
Postpartum endometritis	Anemia
Postpartum sepsis	Death
Air embolism	
Surgical complications	
Recurrence	
'D' factor sensitization	
Death	

(Hibbard, 1988; Green, 1989; Lavery, 1990; Lockwood, 1990; Gilbert and Harmon, 1993; Lockwood, 1994; Konje et al, 1994.)

Pathophysiology

	ABRUPTION	
PARAMETER	**NORMAL PHYSIOLOGY**	**PATHOPHYSIOLOGY**
Spiral arterioles	Intact	Degenerated
Decidua basalis	Intact	Necrosed
Uteroplacental circulation	Closed	Vessel rupture and bleeding
Placental attachment	Complete	Some degree of separation
		Blood may enter myometrium (Couvelaire uterus)
Coagulation and fibrinolysis	Balanced	Retroplacental clot formation
		Thromboplastin release
		DIC
Fetus	Uncompromised	May be acutely or chronically compromised
		IUGR
		Fetal demise
Uterine fundus	Soft	Irritable or rigid

| | PREVIA | |
| | | |

PARAMETER	NORMAL PHYSIOLOGY	PATHOPHYSIOLOGY
Placental implantation	Fundal	Lower segment; may migrate upward
Cervical os	Uncovered	May be partially or completely covered
Placental attachment	Intact	May be partially separated
Vaginal bleeding	None	Mild to moderate
Fetus	Compromised	May be chronically compromised

 Signs & Symptoms

Any or all of the following may be present in placental abruption:

Abdominal discomfort or pain

Back discomfort

Varying degrees of dark vaginal bleeding

Uterine irritability, hypertonia, or rigidity

Shock

Evidence of fetal compromise

(Fox, 1978; Notelovitz et al, 1979; Hurd et al, 1983; Knuppel and Drukker, 1986; Hibbard, 1988; Green, 1989.)

The following are signs and symptoms of placenta previa:

Vaginal bleeding after 20 weeks' gestation

Ultrasonographic evidence of low placental implantation, usually with no pain or uterine activity

 ### *Screening for Appropriateness of Home Care*

After initial stabilization in the acute facility, the patient with one of these placental abnormalities may be considered for home management if certain recommended safety criteria are met:

Stabilization of bleeding (no copious active bleeding in 24 hours)

No evidence of fetal compromise (reassuring NST on day of hospital discharge)

Absence of uterine irritability or contractility

Membranes intact

No evidence of maternal infection

Additionally, the following criteria are recommended:

Patient and support network committed to plan of care

Environment suited to services planned (bedroom and bath on same floor if bed rest ordered, child-care arrangements made)

Realistic expectations on the part of patient and family, including understanding that rehospitalization may become necessary

Distance from hospital appropriate to risk

Home Management

Orders for home care may include the following:
  Bed rest with bathroom privileges
  Regular or high fiber diet (to prevent constipation or straining)
  Skilled nursing visits
  EFS
  Venipuncture for complete blood count (CBC)
  Iron replacement
  Placement of long-life venous catheter for emergency fluid replacement
  Pertinent teaching
Equipment and supplies may include an IV pole, parenteral fluids, and site-care supplies.

Skilled nursing assessment, intervention, and teaching should include the following:

MATERNAL	FETAL
Vital signs	Fundal height
Character and amount of vaginal discharge	FHR
	EFS as ordered
Uterine activity	

Patient Health Teaching

Pertinent health teaching should include the following:
  Activity limits as ordered
  Avoidance of Valsalva maneuver

Dietary adjustments to minimize constipation
or straining at stool (fruit juices, fiber)
Signs and symptoms to report
Abdominal pain
Back pain
Regular contractions
Decreased fetal movement
Small amounts of vaginal bleeding
Signs for which immediate transfer to hospital
is indicated
Uterine rigidity
Significant vaginal bleeding
Signs of shock (pallor, tachycardia,
diaphoresis)
Rupture of membranes
Strong contractions 5 minutes or less apart
Severe perineal pressure

PRETERM LABOR

Definition

Preterm labor is defined as regular uterine contractions with cervical dilation or effacement or rupture of the membranes, occurring between 20 and 37 weeks of gestation (Cunningham et al, 1993; James et al, 1994; Burrow and Ferris, 1995). Uterine contractions without cervical change or membrane rupture are considered uterine irritability or threatened preterm labor (James, 1994).

Incidence

Though the incidence of preterm labor is not well documented, the preterm birth rate is approximately 11% nationwide (March of Dimes, 1993). Up to 83% of neonatal deaths are attributable to prematurity (Bureau of Vital Statistics, 1993).

Etiology

Although the exact mechanism responsible for the initiation of labor has not been fully identified, theories have been advanced regarding the interaction of hormones and their substrates, including prostaglandins, estrogen, progesterone, and oxytocin (Casey and MacDonald, 1986; MacKenzie et al, 1988; Huszar, 1989; Cunningham, 1993).

Risk factors for the development of preterm labor are as follows:

Previous preterm labor
Low socioeconomic status
Poor nutritional status
Substance use (illicit drugs, alcohol, tobacco)

Stress

Other pregnancy complications (placenta previa, placental abruption, preeclampsia, multifetal pregnancy, preterm premature rupture of membranes)

Abdominal surgery or trauma

Chronic disease (diabetes, cardiovascular or renal disease)

Uterine anomalies

Intrauterine, vaginal, fetal, or urinary tract infection

Appendicitis, cholecystitis

(Main and Gabbe, 1987; Morrison, 1990; Gilbert and Harmon, 1993; Burrow and Ferris, 1994.)

Associated Risks

MATERNAL	FETAL AND NEONATAL
Stress related to the threat of premature birth	Intrauterine death
	Side effects of tocolytic agents
	IUGR
Side effects of tocolytic agents	Complications of prematurity: respiratory distress syndrome, intracranial hemorrhage, septicemia, birth trauma, anemia, seizures, long-term neurologic disorders, metabolic disturbances, necrotizing enterocolitis, neonatal death, retinopathy, patent ductus, apnea, bradycardia, poor thermoregulation, sepsis
Infection	

(Escher-Davis et al, 1993; Gilbert and Harmon, 1993; James et al, 1994; Burrow and Ferris, 1995.)

Pathophysiology

As previously stated, labor is probably initiated through a complex interaction of hormones. Prostaglandins (PGE_2 and PGF_2) reliably produce contractions and delivery when used therapeutically (Casey, 1986). Factors that cause irritation of the uterus, including myometrial stretching, sudden decompression, and bacterial invasion, may stimulate the release of prostaglandins. The following table summarizes physiologic alterations:

PARAMETER	NORMAL PHYSIOLOGIC CHANGE	PATHOPHYSIOLOGIC CHANGE
Uterine fundus	Soft	Regular contractions
Cervix	Long, thick, and closed	Some dilation or effacement
Fetal presenting part	Nonengaged or ballot-table	May be engaged

 Signs & Symptoms

The presenting complaints may include the following:

   Low cramplike contractions occurring at regular intervals

   Sensation of pressure over the perineum

   Loss of cervical mucous plug ("bloody show")

The diagnosis of preterm labor, as differentiated from threatened preterm labor or uterine irritability, is made when cervical dilation or effacement is documented.

Screening for Appropriateness of Home Care

The following criteria are recommended before the preterm labor patient is admitted to home care:

- Suggested medical criteria for safety are met:
  - Gestational age between 20 and 36 weeks
  - Cervical dilation less than or equal to 4 cm
  - Fetal membranes intact
  - Successful suppression of contractions for at least 24 hours
- Patient and support network motivated to participate in plan of care
- Environment suited to plan of care and conducive to activity limits ordered (bed, bath, and telephone on same level)

Conversely, the following criteria may suggest that a particular patient is not appropriate for home care:

- Medical safety cannot be established (advanced cervical dilation or bulging membranes), particularly if patient is located a considerable distance from the hospital
- Patient or support network unable or unwilling to participate in plan of care
- Environment unsuited to plan of care

 ## *Home Management*

Orders for assessments and interventions for home care may include the following:

Bed rest with bathroom privileges

Regular diet (may be modified to avoid constipation)

Skilled maternal and fetal assessments

Uterine activity monitoring (electronic or via self-palpation)

Fetal movement counting

EFS: NST, US, or BPP

Medications, including tocolytics, glucocorticoids, or stool softeners

Fluid intake of 2-3 L/day

Pertinent health teaching to patient and support network

NICU video tour

Skilled nursing assessments should include the following:

MATERNAL	
ASSESSMENT	INTERVENTION
Vital signs	Report temperature >101° F orally or apical pulse >120 BPM.
Uterine activity	Report >6 contractions/hr.
Serial cervical examinations	Report progressing dilation or effacement, bulging membranes, or presenting fetal part at ≥3+ station.
Vaginal discharge	Report purulent discharge; transfer to hospital for rupture of membranes.
Urinary system	Report signs and symptoms of UTI.
Subjective symptoms	Report patient complaints of perineal pressure, low abdominal or back cramping, or "bearing down" sensation.

	FETUS
ASSESSMENT	INTERVENTION
FHR	Report FHR <110 BPM or >160 BPM.
Fetal activity	Report decreased fetal movement; transfer to hospital for lack of fetal movement for 4 hours.
Fundal height	Report variation of fundal height 3 cm > or < gestational age in weeks.
NST*	Report reassuring strip.
	Transfer to hospital for nonreassuring strip.
US*	Report results.
BPP*	Report score or results.

*See Appendix 4.

Tocolytic therapy may be employed in the management of preterm labor. Drugs commonly used for this purpose include the following:

Beta-sympathomimetics (ritodrine, terbutaline sulfate)

Magnesium sulfate

Prostaglandin inhibitors (indomethacin)

Calcium channel blockers (nifedipine)

(Gilbert and Harmon, 1993.)

In addition, glucocorticoids (betamethasone, dexamethasone) may be ordered to aid in the maturation of fetal lungs.

Skilled nursing visits should include an assessment of the side effects of the following drugs:

DRUG	SIDE EFFECTS	TOXIC EFFECTS
Beta-sympatomimetics	Mild hypotension	Maternal tachycardia >140 BPM
	Lightheadedness or dizziness	BP <90/60
	Restlessness	Chest pain
	Maternal and fetal tachycardia	Maternal cardiac arrhythmias
	Heart palpitations	Pulmonary edema
	Nausea or vomiting	
Magnesium sulfate	Nausea or vomiting	Respiratory depression
	Diarrhea	Absence of deep tendon reflexes
	Suppression of deep tendon reflexes	
		Severe hypotension
Prostaglandin inhibitors	Nausea	Peptic ulcer
	Diarrhea	Hematuria
	Headache	
	Vertigo or tinnitus	
	Oligohydramnios	
Glucocorticoids	Increased risk of infection	Deep vein thrombosis
	Delayed healing	Electrolyte imbalance
	Exacerbation of diabetes or hypertension	

(Asperheim, 1985; Gilbert and Harmon, 1993; PDR, 1995.)

Patient Health Teaching

Pertinent heath teaching should include information on the following:

Bed rest in left-lateral position

Avoidance of Valsalva maneuver

Dietary adjustments to minimize constipation or straining at stool (fruit juices, fiber)

Signs and symptoms to report
Regular contractions
Perineal pressure
Change in vaginal discharge
Decreased fetal movement
Low back pain or pressure
Change in availability of support network or environment

Signs for which immediate transfer to hospital is indicated
Strong contractions less than 5 minutes apart
Rupture of membranes
Severe perineal pressure
Urge to push

Therapeutic use and side effects of medications as necessary

Use of home monitoring equipment as necessary

It may be helpful to link the preterm labor patient with a "moms on bed rest" telephone support group or to suggest or provide reading material on preterm labor, premature infants, and NICU care.

Visits should be frequent in the first several days of the home care course, then they should be made only as the patient's stability and her knowledge of self-care and reporting parameters allow.

PRETERM PREMATURE RUPTURE OF MEMBRANES

Definition

Preterm premature rupture of the membranes (PPROM) may be defined as a rupture of the fetal membranes before the thirty-seventh week of gestation.

Incidence

Premature rupture of membranes (PROM), a rupture before the onset of labor, occurs in 2% to 18% of all pregnancies; of these instances of PROM, 20% occur before term (Allen, 1991). PPROM results in the onset of labor and preterm delivery in 80% of cases (Williams, 1991). In the remaining 20% of cases, most women go on to deliver within a week.

Etiology

In most cases of PPROM, no direct cause is found. Increased risk of PPROM occurs under the following conditions:

Prior pregnancy complicated by PPROM

Increased intrauterine pressure from multiple gestation or polyhydramnios

Inflammatory reactions due to bacterial invasion, trauma, or placental abnormality

Medical indigence

Nutritional deficiency, particularly zinc

History of multiple amniocenteses or therapeutic abortions

Maternal smoking

(ACOG, 1988; Harger et al, 1990; Sikorski et al, 1990; Allen, 1991; Greenberg and Hankins, 1991.)

Associated Risks

MATERNAL	FETAL AND NEONATAL
Postpartum endometritis	Umbilical cord prolapse or compression
Sepsis	Meconium aspiration syndrome
Death	Pulmonary hypoplasia
Placental abruption	Infection (septicemia, meningitis, pneumonia) after 35 wk
	Prematurity
	Death
	Skeletal compression deformities

(Vintzileos et al, 1987; Goldstein et al, 1989; Ohlsson, 1989; Asrat and Garite, 1991; Cunningham et al, 1993.)

 Pathophysiology

Amniotic fluid is produced continuously throughout pregnancy by the amnion and is breathed, swallowed, and excreted by the fetus. The average volume of fluid is 400 ml at 20 weeks and approximately 1000 ml by term (Brace and Wolf, 1989). If the tear of the membranes is small, it may "heal" spontaneously; if large, amniotic fluid will continue to leak until the fetus is delivered. The average amount of fluid within the uterus depends upon the net loss per day (amount produced minus amount leaked in 24 hours). Though maternal risks associated with PPROM do not vary with the amount of fluid lost, fetal risks do increase in proportion to lost fluid.

PARAMETER	NORMAL PHYSIOLOGIC	PATHOPHYSIOLOGIC CHANGE
Amniotic fluid	400 ml at 20 wk; 1000 ml at term	Varies with net loss; may be <20 ml
Protection from external trauma	Fluid provides optimal cushioning	Loss of optimal cushioning
Protection from bacterial invasion	Membrane provides physical barrier; fluid provides some antimicrobial protection	Loss of physical barrier; decreased antimicrobial action
Fetal physical development	Optimal medium for free movement, aiding symmetrical development	Risk of skeletal compression and deformities
Fetal lung development	Lung expansion and development aided by fetal breathing of fluid	Risk of pulmonary hypoplasia
Umbilical cord	Fluid minimizes risk of entrapment	Risk of cord prolapse or compression
Uterine contractility	Braxton Hicks contractions (benign)	Vastly increased risk of preterm labor, possibly due to sudden decompression leading to inflammatory response and increased prostaglandin production

Signs & Symptoms

Signs of PPROM include either a trickle or sudden gush of fluid from the vagina.

Screening for Appropriateness of Home Care

The following criteria are recommended before the PPROM patient is admitted to home care:

- Suggested medical criteria for safety are met:
  - Gestational age between 20 and 36 weeks
  - Patient and fetus stable for 72 hours
  - No evidence of infection
- Patient and support network motivated to participate in plan of care
- Environment suited to plan of care regarding activity limits and cleanliness

Home Management

Orders for assessments and interventions for home care may include the following:

Bed rest with bathroom privileges

Diet modified to avoid constipation

Skilled maternal and fetal assessments

Uterine activity monitoring

Fetal movement counting

EFS

Medications

Fluid intake of 2-3 L/day

Monitoring and documentation of maternal pulse, FHR, amniotic fluid loss and characteristics, CBC at regular intervals

Pertinent health teaching

NICU video tour

Nursing assessments and interventions should include the following:

MATERNAL	
ASSESSMENT	INTERVENTION
Vital signs	Report oral T >100° F or apical pulse >10 BPM above baseline.
Uterine activity	Report >6 contractions/hour.
	Transfer to hospital for contractions ≤5 minutes apart.
Amniotic fluid loss	Document number of peri pads and their weight every day; document character of fluid.
	Report change in amount of leakage.
	Transfer to hospital for purulence.
Subjective symptoms	Report complaints of perineal pressure or low abdominal or back cramping.
	Transfer to hospital for severe perineal pressure or urge to push.

FETUS	
ASSESSMENT	INTERVENTION
FHR	Report FHR <110 BPM or >10 BPM above baseline.
Fetal activity	Report decreased fetal movement.
Fundal height	Report decrease in 1 week.
NST*	Report reassuring strip to physician.
	Transfer to hospital for nonreassuring strip.
US*	Report results to physician.
BPP*	Report score or results to physician.

*See Appendix 4.

Patient Health Teaching

Pertinent health teaching should include the following:

- Activity limits and positioning as ordered
- Dietary adjustments to prevent straining at stool
- Measurements and documentation of pulse, temperature, fetal movements, amniotic fluid loss
- Signs and symptoms to report
  - Preterm labor
  - Change in character of fluid leaked
  - Temperature greater than 100° F orally
  - Decreased fetal movement
- Signs and symptoms for which immediate transfer to hospital is indicated
  - Contractions 5 minutes or less apart
  - Severe perineal pressure
  - Purulent or meconium-stained fluid
- Medications and equipment use as ordered

GESTATIONAL DIABETES

Definition

Gestational diabetes is defined as "carbohydrate intolerance with onset or first recognition during pregnancy" (Second International Workshop, 1985).

Incidence

Gestational diabetes, more common than preexisting diabetes, occurs in 2% to 3% of pregnant women in the United States (Coustan, 1994). Women at high risk for the development of gestational diabetes are those whose histories include the following:

Family history of diabetes

Stillbirth of unknown etiology

Previous delivery of neonate weighing more than 9 lb

Recurrent spontaneous abortions

Obesity

Hypertensive disorder

Recurrent monilial infection

Polyhydramnios in the absence of fetal anomaly

Glycosuria on two occasions during current pregnancy

(York et al, 1990; Cunningham, 1993; Gilbert and Harmon, 1993.)

Etiology

Pregnancy-related diabetes mellitus occurs in women who have functional defects in pancreatic

B-cells, inhibiting their ability to compensate for the normal insulin resistance of pregnancy *(Hollingsworth and Moore, 1989; Buchanan et al, 1990).*

Associated Risks

Maternal and fetal risks are significantly minimized when control of serum glucose is established and maintained. The risks, directly related to glucose control, are as follows:

MATERNAL	FETAL AND NEONATAL
Spontaneous abortion	Congenital defects
Preeclampsia	Macrosomia
Preterm labor	Delayed lung maturation
Polyhydramnios	Hypoglycemia
Infection	Hyperbilirubinemia
Cesarean section	Polycythemia
Continued diabetes after pregnancy	Placental deterioration in late pregnancy leading to central nervous system (CNS) damage
	Fetal demise

(American Diabetes Association, 1989; Greene et al, 1989; Hollingsworth and Moore, 1989; Stamler et al, 1990; Rosenn et al, 1991; Gilbert and Harmon, 1993; Sibai, 1993; Buchanan and Coustan, 1994.)

Pathophysiology

Parameter	Normal Physiologic Change	Pathophysiologic Change
Fasting maternal glucose level	60-104 mg/dl	≥105 mg/dl
100 g glucose challenge*		
at 1 hr	145-189 mg/dl	≥190 mg/dl
at 2 hr	120-164 mg/dl	≥165 mg/dl
at 3 hr	100-144 mg/dl	≥145 mg/dl
Insulin resistance	Increased	Increased
Insulin production	Increased	Decreased: may lead to hyperglycemia, cellular starvation, metabolic acidosis
Renal function	Intact	Impaired: may lead to vasospasm, preeclampsia, UTI, preterm labor
Fetal development	Intact	Impaired nutrient metabolism: has deleterious effect on organ development
		Fetal hyperglycemia stimulates increased fetal insulin production, causing increased growth and fatty deposits that lead to a large-for-date fetus

*National Diabetes Data Group criteria for abnormal glucose levels

Continued

PARAMETER	NORMAL PHYSIOLOGIC CHANGE	PATHOPHYSIOLOGIC CHANGE
		Resulting macrosomia may lead to birth trauma or asphyxia
		Increased fetal diuresis may lead to polyhdramnios
Placental function	Intact CNS	Impaired: may cause fetal hypoxia, damage, demise
Neonatal metabolism	Intact	Abnormally high insulin production leads to hypoglycemia
Neonatal hematology	Intact	Compensatory increase in production of erythrocytes, increased red cell lysis-hyperbili rubinemia

(American Diabetes Association, 1989; Greene et al, 1989; Hollingsworth and Moore, 1989; Stamler et al, 1990; Rosenn et al, 1991; Gilbert and Harmon, 1993; Sibai, 1993; Buchanan and Coustan, 1994.)

 Signs & Symptoms

The Second International Workshop Conference on Gestational Diabetes recommends screening all pregnant women for gestational diabetes between 24 and 28 weeks of gestation. Signs of hyperglycemia before screening may include the following:

Increased thirst

Increased appetite

Weight loss

Weakness or decreased endurance
Leg cramps
Nausea and vomiting
Pruritus

(American Diabetes Association, 1986; Gilbert and Harmon, 1986; Buchanan and Coustan, 1994.)

 ### Screening for Appropriateness of Home Care

Hospitalization is rarely required for the gestational diabetic patient unless there has been a diabetic crisis such as ketoacidosis. The referral for home care may therefore be generated in the primary provider's office. Screening is geared primarily to the teaching services to be provided. Suggested safety criteria include the following:

Patient and caregiver commitment to the plan of care
Willingness and ability to learn and manage diet regime, blood sugar testing, and insulin administration as needed
Refrigeration for insulin storage

 ### Home Management

Home care orders may include the following:
Skilled nursing visits for assessment and teaching
Glucometer and related supplies
Insulin, syringes, and needles
Specific American Diabetes Association (ADA) diet

Skilled nursing visit assessments, interventions, and teaching should include the following:

ASSESSMENT	INTERVENTION
Blood glucose (BG) levels	Measure BG level using glucometer.
	Report BG ≥200 mg/dl.
	Transfer to hospital for signs and symptoms of ketoacidosis.
	Administer insulin as ordered.
Ketonuria	Report two consecutive positive results.
Fetus	Report FHR <110 BPM or >160 BPM.
	Report fundal height 3 cm >gestational age in weeks.
	Report decreased fetal movement.

Patient Health Teaching

Home care for gestational diabetes may emphasize patient education rather than long-term nursing intervention. Many clinical pathways now in use call for four to six visits with discharge to self-care and primary provider follow-up.

Pertinent health teaching should include instruction on the following:

Teach BG testing at ordered frequency; have patient demonstrate ability to correctly perform test.

Teach diet regime and provide ADA exchange list.

Refer to nutritionist prn.

Teach insulin administration and storage; have patient demonstrate ability to correctly perform procedures.

Teach appropriate sharps disposal.

Teach daily logging of BGs and nutritional intake.

Teach signs and symptoms to report to provider:
Hyperglycemia
Single BG >200 mg/dl
BGs >140 mg/dl three times in 1 week
Illness, particularly if it results in decreased food intake
Decreased fetal movement

MULTIFETAL PREGNANCY

Definition

Multifetal pregnancy, also called multiple gestation, is a pregnancy in which there are two or more fetuses.

Incidence

Spontaneous multifetal pregnancy occurs with the following frequency:

Twins—2 to 3 per 100 pregnancies
Triplets—1 per 7500 pregnancies
Quadruplets—1 per 2,000,000 pregnancies
(Escher-Davis et al, 1990.)

In vitro fertilization and the use of fertility drugs have increased the incidence of multifetal pregnancy over the last 15 years.

Etiology

Monozygotic (identical) twins are the result of the division of the zygote into 2 equal parts, each containing 23 pairs of chromosomes, following fertilization of a single ovum by a single spermatozoon. This may occur in a pregnancy containing twins or, more rarely, in a triplet or quadruplet pregnancy in which two of the fetuses are monozygotic twins and the remainder fraternal siblings. Polyzygotic fetuses are the result of the fertilization of more than one ovum, each with a different spermatozoon.

Associated Risks

A pregnancy of two or more fetuses is associated with increased risk for several pregnancy complications. Overall, the risk of developing some type of complication is approximately 2½ times greater than that of a single gestation. Some of the risks of multifetal pregnancy include the following:

MATERNAL	FETAL AND NEONATAL
Hypertensive disorders	Low birthweight
Hyperemesis gravidarum	Congenital anomalies
Spontaneous abortion	Prematurity
"Vanishing twin" syndrome	Intrauterine demise
Anemia	Stillbirth
Operative delivery	Twin to twin transfusion
Polyhydramnios	"Stuck twin" phenomenon
Antepartum or postpartum hemorrhage	Cord compression
Preterm labor*	Asphyxia
	Fetal entrapment

(Gonen et al, 1990; Cunningham, 1993; Crowther, 1994; O'Grady, 1994.)
*There is evidence in recent literature that the risk of advanced cervical dilation and effacement associated with preterm labor is higher in multifetal pregnancies than in singleton pregnancies because of decreased awareness of uterine contractions caused by increased uterine distension.

Pathophysiology

PARAMETER	NORMAL PHYSIOLOGIC CHANGE	PATHOPHYSIOLOGIC CHANGE
Fundal height	Approximately equal in cm to gestational age in weeks	1.5-2.5 times that of single-ton uterine distension; may lead to preterm labor or postpartum uterine hypotonia and hemorrhage
Cervix	Closed before 36th wk	Stretching of lower segment causes release of prostaglandins; may lead to preterm cervical dilation or effacement
Uterine fundus	Soft, occasional Braxton Hicks contractions	Overdistension may cause irritability; lower segment stretching may cause release of prostaglandins leading to preterm labor
Fetal growth and development	Optimal	Increased risk of suboptimal placental attachment site; decreased transport of nutrients may lead to IUGR
Maternal nutrition	Adequate for needs	Increased HCG levels in 1st trimester may predispose patient to hyperemesis, cellular starvation, central dehydration
Placental or fetal circulation	Optimal	Placental vascular anastomosis may result in twin-to-twin transfusion or increased risk of cord entanglement or compression because of decreased "free space" inside uterus

(Creasy and Resnick, 1989; Gonen et al, 1990; Cunningham, 1993; Crowther, 1994.)

Signs & Symptoms

Early signs that a pregnancy may contain two or more fetuses include the following:

Nausea and vomiting

Fundal height greater than that expected for dates

The diagnosis may be confirmed by ultrasound when suggestion of multifetal pregnancy arises.

 Screening for Appropriateness of Home Care

The primary focus of management is prevention. The patient is to be considered at risk for the development of a pregnancy complication and is to be screened accordingly. Home care may be employed as a method for monitoring and teaching the patient, as well as for providing care when complications occur.

Suggested screening criteria include the following:

Patient and support network understanding of the reason for home care

Motivation to participate in plan of care

Environment suited to intended services (telephone available if home uterine monitoring employed)

 Home Management

Specific home care orders may include the following:

Skilled nursing visits for assessment, intervention, and teaching

Bed rest or limited physical activity

Home uterine monitoring
Serial EFS
Abstinence from intercourse
Tocolytic therapy

Skilled nursing visits should include the following:

Assessment	Intervention
Preeclampsia	Advise bed rest in left-lateral position for hypertension.
Hypertension Proteinuria Edema	Report BP >140/90 and signs of deterioration.
Preterm labor Uterine activity Cervical status	Monitor uterus at home as ordered.
	Conduct serial cervical examinations.
	Administer tocolytic therapy as ordered.
	Report increased uterine activity or cervical changes.
Fetal compromise Fetal movement Fetal heart rates Growth status	Left-lateral positioning.
	Count fetal movements.
	Document FHRs separately ("A," "B," "C") if possible.
	Report EFS as ordered.
	Report decreased fetal movement or nonreassuring NST immediately; report other EFS results per institution policy.
Nutrition and hydration	Increase daily dietary intake by 300 calories per fetus beyond that of singleton pregnancy.
	Administer PO fluids at 3+ L/day.
Coping	Explain rationale for plan of care.
	Encourage patient and family to vent fears and feelings.
	Link with support group.

Patient Health Teaching

Pertinent health teaching should include information on the following:

Activity limits

Caloric intake and fluid needs or nutritional support of multiple fetuses

Signs and symptoms to report

Preterm labor

Decreased fetal movement

Rupture of membranes

Preeclampsia (headache, visual disturbance, periphera edema)

DISSEMINATED INTRAVASCULAR COAGULOPATHY

Definition

Disseminated intravascular coagulopathy (DIC) is massive concurrent intravascular coagulation and fibrinolysis, resulting in the combined threat of thrombosis and hemorrhage (Cunningham, 1993; Duffy, 1994). It occurs after generalized coagulation activity has been triggered (James, 1994).

Incidence

Though the overall incidence of DIC is unknown, it is estimated that severe DIC, resulting in uncontrollable hemorrhaging, occurs in 0.1% of pregnancies (James, 1994).

Etiology

Increased consumption of clotting factors, fibrin, and platelets combines with coagulation failure to cause massive maternal hemorrhage (Creasy and Resnick, 1989). The "trigger" of serious health compromise sets off a series of events, including generalized coagulation, with consumption of coagulation factors occurring faster than replacement. This consumption results in depletion of coagulation factors leading to a reactive fibrinolysis and multiorgan system bleeding (Creasy and Resnick, 1989; Young, 1990). Conditions known to increase the risk of DIC include the following:

Placental abruption
Fetal demise
Severe hypertensive disorder
Amniotic fluid embolism
Abdominal trauma
Sepsis or endotoxic shock
(Creasy and Resnick, 1989; James, 1994.)

Associated Risks

MATERNAL	FETAL AND NEONATAL
Hypovolemic shock	Asphyxia
Infection	Death
Transfusion complications	
Anemia	
Death	

(Creasy and Resnick, 1989; Young, 1990; Cunningham, 1993.)

DIC is a highly volatile and potentially fatal disorder that is inappropriate for home management. It is discussed in this text for the purpose of risk-assessment during the course of caring for other pregnancy complications in the home. The home care plan for any pregnant patient with known precipitating factors should include assessment of and patient instruction for the early symptoms of DIC:

Petechiae or ecchymoses
Hematuria
Bleeding at an IV site
Signs of shock
(Young, 1990.)

If any of the above signs are reported by the patient or caregiver or are noted during a visit, the patient should be transferred immediately to the acute-care facility and the primary provider notified promptly.

EMERGENCY DELIVERY

When delivery appears imminent in a high-risk obstetric home care patient, immediate transfer to an acute-care facility is the intervention of choice. However, perinatal home visiting staff should be prepared if it occurs in the home. In this event, the mother and neonate should be transferred to the acute facility as soon after delivery as is safely possible.

Emergency delivery packs should be part of standard "bag supplies" carried by all perinatal community health nurses. These may be purchased commercially prepared or they may be compiled. The authors recommend the following list:

Sterile gloves
Sterile forceps
Scissors
Sterile water
Bulb or De Lee suction
Cord clamps
Receiving blankets
Newborn cap

Recommended assessments and interventions are listed below:

BEFORE DELIVERY	
ASSESSMENT	INTERVENTION
Maternal status	Document heart rate, pulse, and blood pressure every 5 minutes during labor.
	Monitor for vaginal bleeding.
Labor progression	Monitor and document frequency, strength, and duration of contractions.
	Encourage pushing when presenting part is visible on the perineum.
Fetal status	Auscultate and document FHR every 5 minutes.
	Document fetal movement.
	Monitor for and document meconium-stained amniotic fluid.

AFTER DELIVERY	
ASSESSMENT	**INTERVENTION**
Neonatal status	Assign Apgar scores at 1 and 5 minutes: 0 to 2 points each for color, tone, respiratory effort, heart rate, and response to stimuli.
	Monitor and document neonatal vital signs every 5 minutes.
	Monitor color as continuously as possible.
	Resuscitate as necessary.
	Clamp and cut cord, reserve placenta in plastic bag, or wrap placenta with baby if cord not cut.
Thermoregulation	Place skin-to-skin with mother and cover with receiving blanket if fetal status permits.
	Take and document temperature every 5 minutes.
Maternal status	Monitor and document maternal vital signs as soon as possible after delivery, then repeat after 15 minutes.
	Massage fundus until firm, repeating as necessary.
	Place baby to breast if status permits.
	Use Trendelenburg position for excessive bleeding or signs of shock.

The intended audience for this handbook should note that an unplanned home delivery may include a compromised neonate. CHNs faced with this situation should remain alert for the following signs of neonatal compromise and intervene as appropriate:

Circumoral or central cyanosis

Respiratory rate less than 40 or greater than 60 breaths per minute

Heart rate less than 110 or greater than 160 BPM

Inspiratory retractions

Expiratory grunting

Chapter 3

Home Management of Pregnancy in the Presence of Underlying Disease

CARDIAC DISEASE

Definition

Cardiac disease is defined as any structural or functional pathologic abnormality of the heart that negatively affects cardiac function.

Incidence

Cardiac disease is present in 0.5% to 2.0% of pregnant women, with rheumatic fever responsible for 50% of cardiac disease cases in pregnancy.

Etiology

Cardiac diseases include those of congenital and developmental origin, such as mitral valve prolapse and ventricular septal defect, and they also include cardiomyopathies, such as congestive heart failure (CHF) and coronary artery disease.

Associated Risks

Maternal risks vary with the severity of disease and its effect on the patient's ability to compensate for the added demands of pregnancy. Creasy and Resnick (1989) have defined the maternal cardiac disease risk groups as follows:

GROUP I MORTALITY 1%	GROUP II MORTALITY 5%-15%	GROUP III MORTALITY 25%-50%
Corrected tetralogy of Fallot	Mitral stenosis with atrial fibrillation	Aortic coarctation (complicated)
Pulmonic or tricuspid disease	Artificial heart valves	Myocardial infarction
Mitral stenosis (classes I and II)	Mitral stenosis (classes III and IV)	Marfan's syndrome
Patent ductus	Uncorrected tetralogy	True cardio-myopathy
Ventricular septal defect	Aortic coarctation (complicated)	Pulmonary hypertension
Atrial septal defect		
Porcine valve		

Fetal and neonatal risks include the following:
 Spontaneous abortion in early pregnancy
 CNS hypoxia
 IUGR
 Prematurity
 Death
(Niswander et al, 1967; Ueland et al, 1972; Gilbert and Harmon, 1993; Ueland, 1994.)

Pathophysiology

Parameter	Normal Physiologic Change	Pathophysiologic Change
Blood volume	Increased by 45%	Increased by 45%
Stroke volume	Increased	Decreased due to impaired contractility
Heart rate	Increased by 10-15 BPM	Increased in proportion to decreased stroke volume; inability to compensate leads to cardiac failure
Cardiac output (rate × stroke volume)	Increased by 1.5 L/min	Potential inability to increase enough to meet pregnancy demands
Diastolic filling pressure	Optimal	May be decreased
Systemic vascular resistance	Decreased	May be increased, leading to pulmonary hypertension

(Ueland, 1989; Dennison, 1990; Jelsema and Cotton, 1994; Ueland, 1994.)

 Signs & Symptoms

Severity of compromise is defined symptomatically as follows:

Class I   No limit on physical activity; asymptomatic with ordinary activity

Class II   Slight limit on physical activity; fatigue, dyspnea, palpitations, or chest pain present with ordinary activity

Class III   Marked limit on physical activity; less than ordinary activity results in fatigue, dyspnea, palpitations, or chest pain

Class IV   Inability to perform any physical activity; symptomatic at rest

Progression from a lower to a higher classification indicates functional deterioration (Niswander, 1967; Ueland, 1994).

Screening for Appropriateness of Home Care

For the purpose of medical safety the authors recommend a policy of exclusion for those patients in Class III and Class IV (see previous table). In addition, the following criteria are recommended:

Disease stability (no evidence of progression into excluded risk group or symptomatic class)

Patient and support network commitment to plan of care

Environment conducive to services to be provided

Home Management

Orders for home care may be rendered by the patient's primary obstetric provider, though they may be made in concert with a cardiologist. These orders may include the following:

Skilled nursing visits

Activity limitation or bed rest

Medications as ordered (anticoagulant, diuretic, cardiac glycoside, tocolytic, antihypertensive, stool softening, antiarrythmia drugs)

Low salt diet and/or fluid restriction

Skilled nursing visits should include the following:

Assessment	Intervention

Maternal cardiovascular status
   Vital signs
   Chest pain
   Arrhythmia
   Thrombosis
   Apical and radial pulses
   Edema
	Administer cardiac medications as ordered (anticoagulants, diuretics, or antihypertensives).
	Report hypertension, apical heart rate >120 BPM, chest pain, arrhythmia, positive Homan's sign, apical and radial differences, or increased edema.
	Limit activity as ordered.
	Restrict salt or fluid as ordered.
	Transfer patient to acute facility when signs of acute cardiac failure are present.

Maternal pulmonary status
   Decreased endurance
   Lung sounds
	Report increased dyspnea, adventitious lung sounds, or cough.

Pregnancy integrity Preterm labor	Administer tocolytic and stool softeners as ordered. Monitor uterine activity as ordered. Report uterine contractility, rupture of membranes, or cervical changes. Transfer to hospital when established labor is present.

Fetal status
   Fundal height
   FHR
   Fetal movement
	Report EFS parameters as ordered.
	Report fundal height 3 cm < gestational age in weeks, FHR <110 BPM or >160 BPM, or decreased fetal movement.
	Transfer to hospital for nonreassuring NST or absence of fetal movement.

Patient Health Teaching

Pertinent health teaching should include instruction on the following:

Pathophysiology and plan of care

Activity limitations, diet and fluid orders, medication compliance

Signs and symptoms to report

Generalized edema

Neck vein distension

Respiratory difficulty

Chest pain

Heart palpitations

Sudden weight gain

Increased uterine contractions

Rupture of membranes

Decreased fetal movement

RENAL DISEASE

Definition

Primary renal diseases range from mild forms, such as uncomplicated UTI, to severe forms, such as acute renal failure.

Incidence

UTI occurs at the same rate (2%-10%) in both the pregnant and nonpregnant population (Creasy and Resnick, 1989). Approximately 30% of cases will develop into pyelonephritis if untreated (Whalley, 1967).

Etiology

Disease	Cause
Renal calculi	Calcium deposit, uric acid precipitation
Glomerulonephritis	Bacterial invasion of the renal pelvis
Diabetic nephropathy	Renal disease associated with diabetes mellitus*
Polycystic kidney disease	Metabolic error (congenital)
Renal failure	Acute tubular necrosis, renal cortical
Necrosis, obstructive uropathy	
End stage renal disease	Extensive tubular or renal cortical necrosis

(Creasy and Resnick, 1989; Cunningham, 1993; Lindheimer and Katz, 1994; Paller, 1994.)
*See information on Type I diabetes found later in this chapter in "Endocrine Disorders" section.

Associated Risks

MATERNAL	FETAL AND NEONATAL
Hypertension	Spontaneous abortion
Preeclampsia	Stillbirth
Proteinuria	Neonatal death
Nephrotic syndrome	Prematurity
Decreased renal function	IUGR

(Creasy and Resnick, 1989; Paller, 1994.)

 ## Pathophysiology

PARAMETER	NORMAL PHYSIOLOGIC CHANGE	PATHOPHYSIOLOGIC CHANGE
Glomerular filtration rate	Increased 50%	May be impaired
Serum creatinine level	≤0.8 mg/dl	>0.8 mg/dl
Blood urea nitrogen (BUN) level	5-12 mg/dl	≥13 mg/dl
Bladder tone	Decreased	May be spasmodic in presence of bacterial infection
Blood pressure	Slightly decreased	May be increased
Serum electrolytes	Slightly decreased	May be outside normal range
Urinary output	1.5-3.0 L/day	Potential oliguria
Proteinuria	Negative to trace	≥1+
pH balance	Unchanged from nonpregnant state	Potential metabolic acidosis

(Cunningham et al, 1993; Gilbert and Harmon, 1993; Burrow and Ferris, 1994; Paller, 1994.)

Signs & Symptoms

UTI	Urinary frequency, pain during urination, urgency, suprapubic pressure or pain
Pyelonephritis	Fever, chills, flank pain, malaise
Chronic renal disease	Hypertension, systemic or pulmonary edema, preeclampsia, proteinuria, electrolyte imbalance, decreased urinary output, urine concentration, urticaria, metabolic acidosis

 Screening for Appropriateness of Home Care

Safety criteria vary with the severity of the disease and the services to be provided. For example, for patients with superimposed preeclampsia, the authors recommend following the criteria presented in the discussion of preeclampsia in Chapter 2. In general, the following guidelines are suggested:

Medical stability (no evidence of significant disease progression before discharge from an acute facility)

Patient and support network motivated to accept and participate in plan of care

Environment suited to services to be provided (general cleanliness if home peritoneal dialysis is to be used)

 Home Management

Orders may include some or many of the following:

Skilled nursing visits for assessment, intervention, and teaching

Laboratory services
Peritoneal dialysis
EFS
Medications as ordered (antibiotic, antihyperten-
sive, diuretic, electrolyte balance correction)
Renal diet

Skilled nursing visits should include the following:

Assessment	Intervention

Cardiopulmonary system
  Vital signs
  Lung sounds
	Report hypertension, arrhythmia, tachypnea, neck vein distension, adventitious lung sounds, or fever.

Genitourinary system
  Intake and output
  Dipstick U/A
  Signs and symptoms of infection
  Blood chemistries
  Daily weight
	Report oliguria, generalized edema, or severe urine concentration.
	Report increased proteinuria, nitrites, leukocytes, or subjective UTI symptoms.
	Monitor and report BUN and creatinine levels.
	Administer dialysis as ordered.
	Administer medications as ordered.
	Maintain renal diet as ordered.

Electrolytes	Monitor and report electrolyte panels. Report signs and symptoms of:
Potassium	Hyperkalemia—tachycardia, oliguria, abdominal distension, diarrhea Hypokalemia—anorexia, weakness, hypotension
Sodium	Hypernatremia—specific gravity >1.030, signs and symptoms of dehydration, restlessness, seizures

Continued

ASSESSMENT	INTERVENTION
Calcium	Hypercalcemia—lethargy, headache, weakness, anorexia, flank pain
	Hypocalcemia—irritability, muscle twitch, spasms, paresthesia, hypotension, diarrhea, seizures
Metabolic acidosis	Report urine pH <6.0, rapid deep respirations, or decreased level of consciousness.
Fetal status	Report fundal height 3 cm <gestational age in weeks.
Fundal height	
Fetal movement	Report decreased fetal movement.
FHR	Report FHR <110 BPM or >160 BPM.
NST	Report nonreassuring NST immediately.
US	Report US evidence of growth retardation.

Patient Health Teaching

Pertinent health teaching should include the following signs and symptoms to report:

UTI

Preeclampsia

Acute renal failure

Decreased fetal movement

Spontaneous rupture of membranes or vaginal bleeding

Uterine contractions or cramping

Symptoms of electrolyte imbalance or acidosis

PULMONARY DISEASE

Definition

Pulmonary disease is defined as any pathologic condition of the lungs or upper respiratory tract that has a deleterious effect on gas exchange (Thomas, 1985; Weinberger and Weiss, 1994).

Incidence

Asthma is the most common form of pulmonary disease in women of childbearing age and occurs in 1% to 4% of this population (Mabie et al, 1992).

Etiology

The following is a list of known or theorized causes of pulmonary disease in women of child-bearing age:

DISEASE	CAUSE
Asthma Paroxysmal dyspnea	Allergy

Bronchitis or bronchiolitis
  Inflammation of the
  bronchi or bronchioles
	Viral or bacterial infection

Bronchiectasis	Previous bronchial injury from infection causes irreversible dilation of the bronchi
Chronic obstructive pulmonary disease (COPD)	Long-term exposure to respiratory irritants, such as cigarette smoke, coal dust

Continued

DISEASE	CAUSE
Emphysema Chronic bronchitis	Interstitial or alveolar damage caused by previous severe pulmonary infection
Cystic fibrosis Airway obstruction is caused by chronic inflammation and excessive production of respiratory secretions	Genetic disorder
Sarcoidosis Granuloma of lungs and other organs	Unknown
Pneumonia Inflammation of one or more pulmonary lobes	Bacterial or viral infection
Tuberculosis Inflammation of lower respiratory tract	Mycobacterium infection

(Thomas, 1985; Weinberger and Weiss, 1994.)

Associated Risks

MATERNAL	FETAL AND NEONATAL
Hypoxemia	Hypoxemia
Hyperemesis gravidarum	Prematurity
Preeclampsia	Low birthweight
Labor complications	IUGR
Adult respiratory distress syndrome (ARDS)	Death
Premature rupture of membranes	
CHF	
Poor weight gain	
Death	

(Gordon et al, 1970; Bahna 1972; Cohen et al, 1980; Good et al, 1981; Longo, 1987; Perlow et al, 1992.)

Pathophysiology

PARAMETER	NORMAL PHYSIOLOGIC CHANGE	PATHOPHYSIOLOGIC CHANGE
Respiratory rate	Slightly increased	May be significantly increased
Tidal volume	Slightly decreased	May be significantly decreased
Serum pH	Upper side of normal range (7.40 to 7.42)	Possible respiratory acidosis (≤7.35)
Lung compliance	Increased	May be decreased
Maternal oxygenation	Optimal	May be compromised
		Severe compromise may lead to respiratory failure, ARDS, or death
Fetal oxygenation	Optimal	Compromised when maternal Po_2 is ≤50 mm Hg
		May lead to growth retardation, CNS injury, or death

Signs & Symptoms

DISEASE	CLINICAL MANIFESTATION
Asthma	Respiratory distress characterized by increased respiratory effort (particularly on expiration), wheezing, cough
Bronchiectasis	Cough, dyspnea, foul sputum
Bronchitis or bronchiolitis	Frequent cough (possibly painful), fever, malaise, mucopurulent sputum
COPD	Increased respiratory rate, wheezing, copiously productive cough, frequent respiratory infections
Cystic fibrosis	Chronic respiratory inflammation with cough, dyspnea, and thick, copious respiratory secretions
Sarcoidosis	Granuloma formation in the lungs may cause dyspnea (particularly on exertion) and cough
Pneumonia	Dyspnea, tachypnea, productive painful cough, malaise, fever, shaking chills
Tuberculosis	Dry or minimally productive cough, low-grade fever, malaise; may later cause necrosis, abscesses, fibrosis, and calcification

(Taylor, 1985; Weinberger and Weiss, 1994.)

 Screening for Appropriateness of Home Care

The safety criteria for admission of a pregnant patient with primary pulmonary disease focus on the safety not only of the patient and fetus but also on the safety of others who may be in contact with the patient who has an infectious disease.

Suggested guidelines include the following:
  Patient and her support network motivated to participate in the plan of care
  General cleanliness of the home
  Environment suited to rest, activity limits ordered, respiratory precautions as needed

Home Management

Home care orders may include the following:
  Skilled nursing visits for assessment, intervention, and teaching
  Laboratory services
  EFS
  Bed rest or limited activity
  Increased PO fluids
  Medications (bronchodilators, antibiotics)

Skilled nursing visits should include the following:

Assessment	Intervention
Maternal pulmonary status	Monitor activity as ordered.
Respiratory rate or effort	Increase PO fluids to 2-3 L/day.
Lung sounds	Administer bronchodilators or antibiotics as ordered.
	Conduct chest physiotherapy as ordered.
Sputum	Report increased respiratory distress, failure to respond to medical therapy, change in sputum to purulence, or new adventitious lung sounds.

Continued

Assessment	Intervention
Pregnancy integrity	Administer medications to prevent or treat preterm labor as ordered.
Uterine activity	Monitor home uterine output as ordered.
Serial cervical exams Membrane status	Report increased uterine activity, cervical change, or rupture of membranes.
Fetal status	Administer US or NST with reports as ordered.
Fundal height FHR Fetal movement	Report fundal height 3 cm < gestational age in weeks, FHR <110 BPM or >160 BPM, or decreased fetal movement.
Coping Anxiety	Encourage venting of fears and feelings.
Cooperation with plan of care	Establish multidisciplinary care conferencing that includes patient and caregiver.

Patient Health Teaching

Pertinent health teaching should include the following:

Pathophysiologic condition of disease

Explanation of plan of care (visit schedule, medications, assessments, interventions)

Role of caregiver and support network

Respiratory precautions if applicable (exposure to pathogens and respiratory irritants, disposal of tissues, proper handwashing)

Signs and symptoms to report
  Increased respiratory distress
  Decreased endurance
  T greater than 101° F
  Change in sputum to yellow or green
  Uterine contractions, perineal pressure, or
    rupture of membranes
  Decreased fetal movement

CONNECTIVE TISSUE DISORDERS

Definition

Connective tissue disorders are a group of diseases that affect the connective structures (joints, nerves, blood vessels) and have certain pathologic features in common. These include area-specific or generalized inflammation and in some cases, fibroid deposits (Thomas et al, 1985).

Management of pregnancy in the presence of underlying connective tissue disease varies, depending on the specific condition and its severity. These diseases are not pregnancy complications themselves but rather are considered predisposing factors. This section will not include specific assessments and interventions because of the diversity of possible complications; instead it will focus on identifying pregnancy conditions to which connective tissue diseases predispose. The reader may refer to Chapter 2 for care-planning guidelines.

DISEASE AND DESCRIPTION	IMPLICATIONS FOR PREGNANCY
Rheumatoid arthritis Synovial joint inflammation	May manifest systemically with a predisposition to hypertension, cardiac output deficiency, or thrombosis
Myasthenia gravis Neuromuscular junction disorder	Magnesium sulfate (MgSO4) contraindicated for treatment of preterm labor
Multiple sclerosis Autoimmune demyelination syndrome	No associated threats to fetus; added weight of pregnancy may predispose wheelchair-bound patients to development of multiple sclerosis
Myotonic muscular dystrophy Inherited systemic dystrophy of skeletal and smooth muscle	Increased risk of spontaneous abortion, preterm labor, postpartum hemorrhage, polyhydramnios, congenital defects, neonatal respiratory distress
Polymyositis Systemic inflammation of proximal limb and trunk musculature	Increased risk of spontaneous abortion and stillbirth
Scleroderma Vascular inflammation	Vasospasm and arteriole inflammation with a predisposition to preeclampsia and fetal stress

BLOOD DYSCRASIAS

Definition

Blood dyscrasia is a general term referring to hematologic diseases including anemias and other disorders of blood and its components.

Incidence

The most common form of blood dyscrasia in pregnancy is anemia, most commonly caused by red cell deficiency associated with iron depletion (Horn, 1988).

Etiology

Hematologic disorders in pregnancy and their causes are listed as follows:

DISORDER	CAUSE OR DESCRIPTION
Anemia	
Iron deficiency	Iron store depletion or poor intake
Folate deficiency	Inadequate intake of folic acid
Vitamin B_{12} deficiency	Addison's disease, tropical sprue
Bone marrow aplasia	Failure of erythrocyte formation
Malignancies	
Leukemia (acute)	Malignant proliferation of immature cells
Leukemia (chronic)	Malignant excessive granulocyte formation

Continued

Disorder	Cause or Description
Hodgkin's disease	Malignant lymphatic disease
Non-Hodgkin's lymphomas	Malignant lymphatic disease
Hemoglobinopathies	Inherited globin synthesis or structural anomaly
Thalassemia syndromes	
Beta	Inherited defect in production of beta hemoglobin
Alpha	Inherited defect in production of alpha hemoglobin
Major	Homozygous—symptomatic (alpha or beta)
Minor	Heterozygous—asymptomatic carrier (alpha or beta)
Sickle cell syndromes	Inherited structural variant of globin chain-producing sickle-shaped erythrocytes impairing oxygen-carrying capacity
Disease	Homozygous—symptomatic
Trait	Heterozygous—asymptomatic
Crisis	Acute impairment of oxygen transport in sickle cell disease, causing capillary flow obstruction
Thrombocytopenia	Preeclampsia, HELLP syndrome, idiopathic decrease in platelet count
Thrombocytopenic or hemolytic uremic syndrome	Platelet thrombi in the microcirculation

(Thomas et al, 1985; Duffy, 1994; Letsky et al, 1994.)

Associated Risks

MATERNAL	FETAL AND NEONATAL
Fatigue	IUGR
Joint pain	Prematurity
Pica	Low birthweight
Cardiac failure	Hemolytic disease of the newborn (HDN)
Liver or spleen enlargement	Hydrops fetalis
Rh sensitization	Kernicterus
Disseminated intravascular coagulopathy	Fetal demise or neonatal death
Renal damage or failure	
Hemorrhage	
Side effects related to chemotherapeutic agents	
Death	

(Romero et al, 1985; Chamberlain, 1991; Horner et al, 1991; Sibai, 1991; Sargeant, 1992; VanEnck et al, 1992; Cunningham et al, 1993; Duffy, 1994.)

Patient Health Teaching

Pertinent health teaching should include the following:

Activity and diet as ordered

Signs and symptoms to report

Change in urinary habits

Bleeding

Medication toxicity

Signs for which immediate transfer to hospital
   is indicated
   DIC
   Vaginal hemorrhage
   Extreme weakness or fatigue
   Respiratory difficulty

ENDOCRINE DISORDERS

Definition

Endocrine disorder is a term used to reflect the hypo- or hyperfunctional state of any of the endocrine glands. This section highlights dysfunction of the pancreas and thyroid, the two most common endocrine disorders affecting women of childbearing age.

Incidence

Preexisting diabetes mellitus occurs in approximately 2% of the pregnant population (Chamberlain, 1991). Hyperthyroidism (Graves' disease) affects 0.2% of the pregnant population (Mestman, 1994).

Etiology

Diabetes is a carbohydrate metabolism disorder caused by failure of the pancreatic beta cells to secrete sufficient insulin because of genetic factors, trauma, or acquired disease of the pancreas (Thomason, 1981). Hyperthyroidism (Graves' disease) is overproduction of thyroid hormone, caused by genetic factors, toxicity, carcinoma, or thyroiditis, resulting in an increased metabolic rate (Thomas, 1981; Metsman, 1994).

Associated Risks

DIABETES MELLITUS	HYPERTHYROIDISM
Maternal vascular disease	Pyelonephritis
Spontaneous abortion	Anemia
Preeclampsia	Hypertension
Preterm labor	Amnionitis
Polyhydramnios	CHF
Instrumental delivery	Thyroid crisis (thyroid storm)
Ketoacidosis	Neonatal hyperthyroidism
Fetal and neonatal hypo- or hyperglycemia	Spontaneous abortion
	Stillbirth
Congenital defects	Neonatal death
Macrosomia	Fetal goiter
Delayed lung maturity	Congenital anomalies
Neonatal hyperbilirubinemia	
Neonatal polycythemia	
Prematurity	
Fetal and neonatal death	

(Mestman, 1981; Zakarija et al, 1983; Cooper, 1985; Greene et al, 1989; Hollingsworth and Moore, 1989; Garner et al, 1990; Stamler et al, 1990; Rosenn et al, 1991; Buchanan and Coustan, 1994; Gabbe, 1994; Mestman, 1994.)

Pathophysiology

DIABETES MELLITUS		
PARAMETER	NORMAL PHYSIOLOGIC CHANGE	PATHOPHYSIOLOGIC CHANGE
Insulin production	Increased with demand	Suboptimal
Insulin resistance	Increased (diabetogenic state)	Increased
Fasting blood sugar level	60-105 mg/dl	>105 mg/dl Poor metabolic control may lead to maternal renal damage, vascular disease, retinopathy, neuropathy, fetal macrosomia, and CNS damage or fetal wastage caused by placental deterioration.

(National Diabetes Data Group, 1989.)

HYPERTHYROIDISM		
PARAMETER	NORMAL PHYSIOLOGIC CHANGE	PATHOPHYSIOLOGIC CHANGE
Total thyroxine (T_4) level	10-17 mcg/dl	>17 mcg/dl
Free T_4 level	1-2 ng/dl	>2 ng/dl significant increase may lead to pyelonephritis, anemia, preeclampsia, amnionitis; if untreated, may

Continued

	HYPERTHYROIDISM	
PARAMETER	**NORMAL PHYSIOLOGIC CHANGE**	**PATHOPHYSIOLOGIC CHANGE**
		lead to preterm labor, spontaneous abortion, or maternal or fetal sepsis after trauma; infection may lead to thyroid storm or crisis (potentially fatal)
Basal metabolic rate	Slightly increased	Moderately to profoundly increased
(T, pulse, respiration)		Generalized hyper-thermia
		Nervousness
		Tremor
		Tachycardia
		Tachypnea
		Increased food intake in thyrotoxicosis; may include weight loss or insomnia
Neck examination	Within normal limits	Goiter
Eye examination	Within normal limits	Potential for:
		Exophthalmos
		Photophobia
		Frequent tearing
		Periorbital swelling
Fetal status	Normal growth and development	IUGR, neonatal hyperthyroidism, low birthweight, severe hypermetabolic symptoms (rare)

(Fisher, 1976; Cove and Johnson, 1985; Mestman, 1994; Burrow and Ferris, 1994.)

Home Management

Diabetes mellitus

Home management of diabetes, as discussed in Chapter 2, centers around teaching the patient to be independent in such tasks as testing blood sugar, monitoring diet, and reporting potential danger signs. Home management of preexisting diabetes, particularly Type I (insulin-dependent), focuses on reinforcing the patient's knowledge about the disease, teaching her about diabetes as it relates to pregnancy, keeping blood sugar and weight under tight control, and closely monitoring the maternal and fetal status. Typical orders may include the following:

    Skilled nursing visits for assessment, intervention, and teaching

    Frequent blood sugar testing

    EFS

    Nutritionist consult

Skilled nursing visits should include the following:

ASSESSMENT	INTERVENTION
Serum glucose	Teach blood sugar testing at least 4 times per day (before each meal and at bedtime).
	Teach correct dosing, storage, and administration of insulin (may be sliding scale).

Continued

Assessment	Intervention
	Teach logging of blood sugar levels, diet, daily weight, and medications.

Maternal status
  Vital signs
  Signs and
  symptoms of
  infection
	Report signs and symptoms of infection: T >101° F, urinary symptoms, signs of vaginal infection, renal involvement, or breakdown of skin integrity.

	Report decreased urinary output, hypertension, or flank pain.
	Teach routine skin inspections; report breakdown.
Pregnancy integrity Uterine activity	Report signs and symptoms of preterm labor or membrane rupture.
Polyhydramnios	Report uterine overdistension.
Fetal status	Report fundal height deviation >3 cm from gestational age in weeks.
	Report FHR <110 BPM or >160 BPM.
	Teach fetal movement counting; report decrease or absence.
	Report EFS parameters as ordered.

Patient Health Teaching

Pertinent health teaching should include the following:

Review of blood sugar testing technique, accurate recording

Instruction of specific ADA diet

Daily review of weights

Review of insulin dosing, storage, and administration technique

Signs and symptoms to report
  Hypo- or hyperglycemia
  Viral or bacterial infection
  Decreased fetal movement
  Decreased food intake caused by illness
  Blood sugar outside primary care provider's
    ordered parameters
  Skin breakdown
  Visual or neurologic symptoms
  Signs of renal involvement
  Signs of preeclampsia
  Uterine contractions, perineal pressure, or
    rupture of membranes

Hyperthyroidism

Management of hyperthyroidism focuses on maintaining thyroid hormone levels within the appropriate range through frequent testing and medication. The role of the CHN is largely one of teaching.

  Orders may include the following:
  Skilled nursing visits for assessment, intervention, and teaching
  Laboratory services for hormone level testing
  EFS

Skilled nursing visits should include the following:

ASSESSMENT	INTERVENTION
Thyroid hormone level	Teach compliance with testing regimen.
	Report level outside ordered parameters.
Maternal status	Report hyperactivity, insomnia,
Thyrotoxicosis	hyperthermia, weight loss, or tremor.
Cardiopulmonary	Report signs and symptoms of CHF.
Urinary tract	Report signs and symptoms of UTI or renal involvement.
	Transfer to acute facility immediately for evidence of thyroid storm:
	Abrupt onset of fever
	Diaphoresis
	Tachycardia
	Pulmonary edema
	Restlessness
Fetal status	Report fundal height deviation >3 cm
Fundal height	from gestational age in weeks.
FHR	Report FHR <110 BPM or >160 BPM.
Fetal activity	Report decreased or absent fetal movement.
	Report EFS parameters as ordered.

Patient Health Teaching

Pertinent health teaching should include the following:

Explanation of the disease and its management in pregnancy

Importance of compliance with hormonal level
  testing and medication regimen
Signs and symptoms to report
  Restlessness, tremors, or jitters
  Headache or visual disturbances
  Decreased or absent fetal movement
  Abnormal vaginal discharge, fever, or lower
    abdominal pain
  Signs of UTI and kidney infection
Signs for which the patient should immedi-
  ately go to the hospital
  Sudden fever
  Sweating
  Respiratory difficulty
  Restlessness

SUBSTANCE ABUSE

Definition

The term **drug abuse** is defined in *Mosby's Medical, Nursing, & Allied Health Dictionary* as "the use of a drug for a nontherapeutic effect, especially one for which it was not prescribed or intended." The term **drugs** in this section is used to refer to any substance that has the potential for abuse and is used to affect consciousness, mood, and perception.

Incidence

Chemical dependency among women of childbearing age is a significant problem. Data from the National Household Survey on Drug Abuse in 1990 illustrate the scope of the problem as shown in Tables 3-1 and 3-2.

TABLE 3-1   Drug use among women aged 15 to 44 years

SAMPLE SIZE	3522
% having used any illegal drug in	
Lifetime	48.5
Past year	17.3
Past month	8.0

TABLE 3-2   Drug use in past month among women aged 15 to 44 years

Alcohol	30.5*
Marijuana	3.9*
Cocaine	0.5*

(National Institute on Drug Abuse, 1990.)
*In millions.

Etiology

The etiology of substance abuse may have several factors, including the following:

Familial tendency

Peer pressure

Depression

Other psychosocial factors

Associated Risks

MATERNAL	FETAL AND NEONATAL
Malnutrition	IUGR
Addiction	Addiction
Withdrawal syndrome	Withdrawal syndrome
Placental abruption	Prematurity
Preterm labor	Congenital anomalies
Sexually transmitted diseases	Congenital infection
	Respiratory distress syndrome
Overdose	Intrauterine demise
Myocardial ischemia	Neonatal death
Intracerebral hemorrhage	Developmental delay
Coma	Cerebral hemorrhage
Death	Sudden infant death syndrome
	Seizures

(Chasnoff et al, 1985; Mercado et al, 1989; Mastrogiannis et al, 1990; Woods and Plessinger, 1990; Chasnoff, 1991; Hurd et al, 1991; Gazaway, 1994; Lee, 1994; Welch and Sokol, 1994.)

Pathophysiology

PARAMETER	NORMAL PHYSIOLOGIC CHANGE	PATHOPHYSIOLOGIC CHANGE
Maternal self-care	Optimal	Late or no registration for prenatal care; poor hygiene with predisposition to infection, exposure to human immunodeficiency virus (HIV), hepatitis, tuberculosis (TB)
Nutrition	Increased to 2500 kcal/day	Impaired nutrient absorption or poor food intake that may lead to malnutrition, IUGR
Cardiovascular	Blood volume and cardiac output increases; peripheral vascular resistance decreases	Labile hypertension and vasospasm that may lead to: Hypertensive crisis Cardiac arrhythmias Cardiomyopathy Ruptured aneurysm Myocardial infarction
Pulmonary	Respiratory rate increases to meet pregnancy demands	Chronic rhinitis, pulmonary edema, pneumothorax caused by airway irritation
CNS	Optimal	Cerebral vasospasm and capillary leakage that may lead to hemorrhage or seizures, coma, death

Continued

Parameter	Normal Physiologic Change	Pathophysiologic Change
Gastrointestinal system	Slowed gastric motility	Gastrointestinal and hepatic ischemia, hepatomegaly and splenomegaly, cirrhosis
Renal system	Increased renal flow	Renal insufficiency and GFR creatinine levels that may lead to toxic BUN and acute renal failure
Reproductive system	Increased uterine size and vascularity	Uterine ischemia and decreased uteroplacental flow that may lead to infarct, placental insufficiency, umbilical vasospasm, hence spontaneous abortion, placental abruption, preterm labor
		Lifestyle choices that cause predisposition to sexually transmitted diseases
Fetus	Optimal growth and development	Malnutrition and placental ischemia that may lead to IUGR; systemic vasospasm that may lead to cerebral hemorrhage or infarct and seizures; placental abruption that may lead to anemia, CNS insult or death, prematurity, and related complications

Screening for Appropriateness of Home Care

Home care referrals for the addicted pregnant patient may be generated by the primary care provider or the substance abuse treatment center. Home management for this type of problem, unlike for other diseases or complications, is required not because the patient is homebound but rather because the home setting is the optimal place for rendering services and for assessing lifestyle adaptations. Suggested screening criteria include the following:

> Motivation of the patient and support network to participate in the plan of care
> Completion of detoxification process
> Enrollment in a long-term counseling program

Home Management

Orders may include the following:

> Skilled nursing visits for assessment, intervention, teaching, and case management
> Participation in group or individual drug and alcohol counseling
> EFS

Skilled nursing visits should include the following:

Assessment	Intervention

Maternal status
Cardiovascular
  Respiratory
  Liver
  CNS
	Report cardiac arrhythmia, vital signs, adventitious lung sounds, oliguria, jaundice, change in mentation, or hypertension.

Fetal status
  FHR
  Fetal movement
  Fundal height
	Report FHR <110 BPM or >160 BPM.
	Report decreased fetal movement.
	Report fundal height deviation >3 cm from gestational age in weeks.
	Report EFS parameters as ordered.

Addiction
  Subjective history or use
  Signs of current use or withdrawal
  Urine toxicology testing (voluntary)
	Report signs of active drug use or withdrawal.
	Transfer to hospital for overdose.

Coping
  Resources for support system
  Depression or suicidal ideation
	Refer to community support group.
	Encourage participation in care and monitoring process; reward success.
	Provide hotline numbers (1-800-COCAINE).

Patient Health Teaching

Pertinent health teaching should include instruction on the following:

Use of hotline or group sponsor for cravings

Risks associated with alcohol and drug use

Signs and symptoms to report

Hypertensive crisis

Chest pain

Severe headache

Rupture of membranes

Vaginal bleeding or abdominal pain

Uterine contractions

Decreased fetal movement

Chapter 4

Home Support for Perinatal Loss and Grieving

Perinatal-loss grieving develops with the demise of the fetus or newborn *anytime after parental bonding has occurred.*

Support mechanisms offered by home care personnel are based on grief phases as noted (Davis, 1984).

Phase I	Shock and numbness; peaks at 1-2 wk and at 1 yr	Physical manifestations include pain, emptiness, crying, loss of strength, trembling, sleep disturbance, loss of appetite, and acting out anger.
		Emotional responses include disbelief, confusion, restlessness, and helplessness.
		Psychologic responses include egocentrism, preoccupation with the deceased, and distancing self.
Phase II	Searching and yearning; peaks at 2 wk to 4 mo	Physical manifestations include crying, acting out anger, sleeplessness, and change in eating habits; there is a need to talk about events surrounding the loss and the need to look for answers.
		Emotional responses include separation anxiety, conflict, stress, and sense of something sinister.
		Psychologic responses include hypersensitivity, denial, anger and frustration, sense of presence, dreaming, fear, and guilt.

Continued

Phase III	Disorganization and depression; peaks at 4-6 mo	Physical manifestations include weakness, fatigue, increased sleep needs, and depressed immune system.
		Emotional responses include hibernation and obsessional review; there is a need to seek for explanations and to choose to go forward or not.
Phase IV	Reorganization; peaks at 1 yr and ongoing	Physical manifestations include healing, immune restoration, increased energy, return to normal sleep patterns, and normalization of appetite.
		Emotional responses include sense of control, identity, responsibility, and ability to live with what has happened.
		Psychologic responses include forgiveness, forgetting intense pain, desire to help others with similar experience, hope for future, and expectation and preparation for anniversary reactions.

Support immediately after the loss period is designed to provide care for the patient and her family. Basic needs are often neglected during this time and may be provided through the use of community networking. Generally, the parents are NOT receptive at this point to support groups because of the intense internalization of their feelings. Health care team members should avoid making referrals for bereavement support just to be able to "do something." Simply making oneself available to listen is often all that is needed.

In Phase II receptivity to bereavement support is high. There is a great need to talk about the experience to make sense of it. During this time there may also be some effort at scapegoating to deal with anger and frustration. The family may express the fear of attempting another pregnancy; counseling may be offered based upon the risk factors involved. A referral for genetic counseling should be made as merited.

At Phase III the parents may wish to "revisit" their memories by contacting the personnel involved. This closes the loop and indicates a healthy resolution response.

Follow up by the primary CHN should include the following:

- Visit in the immediate aftermath of the loss
- Assistance in gathering mementos (lock of hair, photograph, baby blanket, footprint sheet)
- Telephone contact on a regular basis for several weeks
- Notification of the primary provider for evidence of dysfunctional grieving
- Referrals for grief counseling or bereavement support at the appropriate time, including specific groups for sibling counseling
- Provision of grief literature
- Encouragement of spiritual guidance as needed

Chapter 5

Postpartum Home Care for the High-Risk Family

The following represents possible orders for home care management of the postpartum and neonatal patient:

- Skilled nursing visits for assessment, intervention, and teaching
- Laboratory services
- Lactation support
- Wound care
- Durable medical equipment or supplies (dressings, bili lights)
- Coordination of care and case management

Each patient should have an individualized care plan based upon her specific needs; however, generic skilled nursing visits should include the following:

POSTPARTUM CARE

Assessment	Intervention
Vital signs	Report T > 101° F, P >120 or < 60, R >30 or <12 breaths per minute, SBP >140 mm Hg or <90 mm Hg, or DBP > 90 mm Hg or < 50 mm Hg.
Cardiovascular	
Heart rate and rhythm	Report cardiac arrythmia, orthostatic blood pressure changes, + Homans' sign, headache, visual disturbances, edema, or excessive fatigue.
Homans' sign	
Postpartum diuresis	Administer and teach medications as ordered.
	Monitor cardiac functions as ordered.

Continued

Assessment	Intervention
Respiratory	
Respiratory effort	Report dyspnea, tachypnea, adventitious lung sounds, or poor oxygenation.
Lung sounds	Monitor oxygen saturation as ordered.
Endurance	Administer and teach medications as ordered.
Gastrointestinal	
Nutrition	Report signs of malnutrition or anorexia.
Bowel function	Teach adequate nutrition and fluids.
	Teach therapy for constipation.
Hepatic symptoms	Report jaundice, right upper quadrant pain, or intolerance to fatty foods.
Urologic	
Amount and character of urine	Report signs and symptoms of UTI or acute renal failure.
Flank pain	
Reproductive	
Fundus	Teach self-fundal assessment and massage.
Lochia	Report signs of postpartum hemorrhage or infection.
	Teach periincision care.
Breasts	
Engorgement	Teach breast care and milk expression and storage.
Milk production	Teach adequate fluid intake.
	Report signs and symptoms of mastitis.
Hematologic	
Hematocrit	Replace iron as ordered.
Hemoglobin	Report laboratory results.
Endocrine	
Diabetes	Review and monitor blood sugar testing.

Continued

ASSESSMENT	INTERVENTION
Hyperthy-roidism	Review and monitor thyroid hormone level.
Hypothy-roidism	Report results outside parameters or diabetic or thyroid crisis.
	Report depression, diarrhea, or fatigue.
Neurologic	
Level of conscious-ness	Report change in mentation, syncope, significant depression, seizure, or abnormal deep tendon reflexes.
Affect	
Seizure	
Reflexes	
Psychosocial	
Coping	Refer to support services as needed for parenting instruction, teen-mother support, drug or alcohol abuse, or domestic violence.
Support network	
Financial status	
	Encourage venting of fears and feelings.
	Refer to Department of Social Services for financial or food assistance as needed.
	Coordinate care with other services.
Knowledge deficit	Teach self-care of periincision and breasts.
	Provide lactation support and teaching.
	Refer to support group as necessary for such things as twins or premature infant.
	Report signs and symptoms including:
	Bright red, heavy vaginal bleeding
	Signs of wound infection (redness, warmth, swelling, purulent drainage)
	Signs of endometritis (fever, chills, lower abdominal pain, purulent vaginal discharge)
	Danger signals particular to individual disease process

NEONATAL CARE

Assessment	Intervention
Vital signs	Report axillary T > 100° F, AP >160 or <100, or R >60 or <36 breaths per minute.
Skin	
Jaundice	Administer phototherapy as ordered for hyperbilirubinemia.
Turgor	
Cord	Teach cord care.
Surgical incision	Perform and teach wound care. Teach hygiene.
	Report signs and symptoms of infection, unresolving jaundice, or umbilical bleeding.
Cardiovascular	
Heart sounds	Report cardiac arrythmia, signs of cardiac failure, poor peripheral pulses, or systemic edema.
Pulses	
Edema	
	Administer and teach medications as ordered.
Respiratory	
Respiratory rate or effort	Report grunting and nasal flaring or retracting.
Oxygenation	Report cyanosis.
Lung sounds	Monitor pulse oximetry as ordered.
	Administer and teach medications as ordered.
Gastrointestinal	
Weight each visit	Teach infant feeding, burping, and reflux precautions as ordered.
Nutritional status	Teach relief of constipation by such means as water and rectal stimulation as ordered.

Continued

ASSESSMENT	INTERVENTION
Bowel function Abdominal girth or tenderness	Report significant increase in abdominal girth or apparent abdominal tenderness or absence of stool for 3 days.
Projectile vomiting	Report feeding difficulties or signs and symptoms of malnutrition or dehydration.
Hydration Feeding history	Teach formula preparation and storage as indicated.
Genitourinary	
Voiding	Report decreased urinary output.
Circumcision	Report signs and symptoms of circumcision infection or hemorrhage.
	Teach perineal and circumcision care.
Neuromuscular	
Affect	Report irritability or lethargy.
Tone Newborn reflexes	Report hyper- or hypotonia and abnormal deep tendon reflexes.
	Report poor root or suck or swallow.
Head circumference and cranial sutures	Report significant increase in head circumference, widening cranial sutures, or seizure activity.
Sleeping patterns Seizures	Teach infant safety and stimulation.
Psychosocial	
Learning needs	Encourage family to vent feelings.
Safety Environment Bonding	Teach infant care, sleep and hygiene needs, feeding, axillary T, and bathing as necessary.
	Teach childproofing.
	Refer to support or parenting group as needed.

Continued

Assessment	Intervention
	Report signs and symptoms of feeding difficulties, elimination problems, or illness (fever, irritability or lethargy, vomiting, diarrhea).
	Report signs of neglect or abuse to child protective authorities.
	Teach care per specific disease, anomaly, or diagnosis as required.
Growth and development	
Weight gain	Report signs of developmental delay.
Milestones	Teach infant stimulation.
	Enroll in early intervention services as developmental testing requires.

Maternal Assessment Guide

PARAMETER	NORMAL RANGE
Temperature	97.5°-99° F
Heart rate	10-15 beats per minute above prepregnant rate
Status	Strong, steady
Respiratory rate	12-24 breaths per minute
Status	Easy, no adventitious sounds
Blood pressure	Systolic: 90-140 mm Hg Diastolic: 50-80 mm Hg
Deep tendon reflexes	1-2+
Fundus	Soft
Cervix	Long, thick, and closed before week 37
Weight gain	Slow and steady to a maximum of 25-40 lb at term
PO fluid intake (avg/day)	2-3 L
Caloric intake (avg/day)	2200-2600 kcal
Urine output (per 24 hr)	2000-3000 ml

Creasy et al, 1989; Cunningham et al, 1993.

Appendix **2**

Fetal Assessment Guide

PARAMETER	NORMAL RANGE
Fetal heart rate	110-160 beats per minute
Fetal movement	≥4 per hour
Fundal height (cm)	Equal to gestational age in weeks after week 20 (±2 cm)

Cunningham et al, 1993.

Fetal Growth and Development Guide

Gestational Age (weeks)	Length (cm)	Femoral Length (mm)	Biparietal Diameter (mm)	Weight (g)
12	9	11	22	14
16	16	24	36	100
20	25	36	50	300
24	30	47	62	600
26	32.5	52	67	800
28	35	56	72	1001
30	37.5	60	77	1350
32	40	64	82	1675
34	42.5	67	86	2001
36	45	70	90	2340
38	47.5	73	93	2775
40	50	75	96	3250

Sabbagha, 1983.

Electronic Fetal Surveillance Guide

Ultrasound*

Measure and document the following per order:

- gestational age by dates
- length
- biparietal diameter
- femoral length
- amniotic fluid index
- estimated fetal weight
- placental location
- status of internal cervical os
- fetal movement and respirations
- any other specific observations ordered

Record date and time of test, along with patient's name, record number, and status before and after procedure.

Report findings to primary provider.

Send copy of still pictures or video recording to primary provider.

---

*Authors recommend this test be performed only by staff specifically trained for and experienced with the procedure.

*Nonstress Test**

Parameters: ≥3 distinct fetal movements during a 20-minute strip

Reactive: >2 accelerations of 15 beats per minute above baseline lasting at least 15 seconds following each fetal movement

Reassuring short- and long-term variability

Nonreactive: failure to meet reactive criteria

(Gilbert and Harmon, 1993.)

Record date and time of test, along with patient's name, record number, and status before and after procedure.

Report findings to primary provider.

Send copy of strip to primary provider.

---

*Authors recommend this test be performed only by staff specifically trained for and experienced with the procedure.

Common Laboratory Values

TEST	NORMAL
pH	7.35-7.45
Blood urea nitrogen	7-18 mg/100 ml
Creatinine	0.4-1.5 mg/dl
Lecithin to sphingomyelin ratio (L/S)	2:1
Liver enzymes	
SGOT	0-30 IU/L
SPGT	4-24 IU/L
Complete blood count	
WBC	5,000-10,000/mm^3
RBC	3.6-5.0 million/mm^3
Platelets	150,000-350,000/mm^3
Hematocrit	36-48%
Hemoglobin	12-16 g/100 ml
Electrolytes	
Sodium	135-145 mg/dl
Potassium	3.5-5.3 mEq/L
Magnesium	1.3-2.1 mEq/L
Calcium	4.65-5.28 mEq/L
Chloride	98-106 mEq/L
Dipstick urinalysis	
Ketones	Negative
Protein	Negative
Glucose	Negative
WBC	Negative or trace
pH	4.5-8
Specific gravity	1.015-1.025

Sibai, 1991; Cunningham et al, 1993; Fishbach, 1996.

A p p e n d i x **6**   Commonly Prescribed Medications*

NAME	INDICATIONS	DOSAGE†	SIDE EFFECTS
Ritodrine	Used for labor suppression	PO: 10-20 mg q 4-6 hr	Increased maternal and fetal heart rates
Terbutaline	Used for labor suppression	PO: 2.5-5.0 mg q 4-6 hr Continuous subcutaneous pump: 0.05-0.075 mg/hr	Increased maternal and fetal heart rates
Magnesium gluconate	Used for labor suppression	PO: 1.0 g q 2-4 hr	Nausea, vomiting, diarrhea

Ridgeway et al, 1990; Eronen et al, 1991; Gilbert and Harmon, 1993; PDR, 1995.

*The authors and publisher have made every attempt to check dosages and nursing content for accuracy. Because the science of pharmacology is continually advancing, our knowledge base continues to expand. Therefore we recommend that the reader always check product information for changes in dosage or administration before administering any medication. This is particularly important with new or rarely used drugs.

†This dosage information is meant as a general guideline. Individual needs may vary.

Continued

Name	Indications	Dosage	Side Effects
Indomethacin	Used for labor suppression	PO: 25 mg q 4 hr	Oligohydramnios, premature closure of the ductus arteriosus
Nifedipine	Used for labor suppression or as an antihypertensive	PO or SL: 10-20 mg q 3 to 8 hr	Headache, fatigue, hypotension
Glucocorticoids (betamethasone, dexamethasone)	Used to induce fetal lung maturation	Two doses of 12 mg 24 hr apart	Increased infection risk; delayed wound healing
Beta blockers (pindolol, oxprenolol)	Antihypertensive	PO: 10 mg	Anxiety, paresthesias, dyspnea, edema

A p p e n d i x **7**

Human Fetotoxic Chemical Agents

MATERNAL MEDICATION	REPORTED EFFECTS ON FETUS OR NEONATE
ANALGESICS	
Indomethacin (Indocin)	Prolongs gestation (monkey); in neonates, used to close patent ductus arteriosus
Narcotics	70% of maternal level; death, apnea, depression, bradycardia, hypothermia
Salicylates	Death in utero; hemorrhage, methemoglobinemia, albumin-binding capacity, salicylate intoxication, difficult birth, (?) prolonged gestation
ANESTHESIAS	
Conduction	Indirect effect of maternal hypotension; direct effect—convulsions, death, acidosis, bradycardia, myocardial depression, fetal hypotension, methemoglobinemia
Paracervical	Methemoglobinemia, fetal acidosis, bradycardia, neurologic depression, myocordial depression

From Bobak IM, Lowdermilk DL, Jensen MD: *Maternity nursing*, ed 4, St Louis, 1995, Mosby.

Continued

Maternal Medication	Reported Effects on Fetus or Neonate
ANTICOAGULANTS	
Coumarins	Fetal death, hemorrhage, calcifications
ANTICONVULSANT AGENTS	
Barbiturates	Irritability and tremulousness 4 to 5 months after birth, hemorrhage, enzyme inducer
Phenytoin and barbiturate	Congenital malformations, cleft lip and palate, congenital heart disease (CHD), central nervous system (CNS) and skeletal anomalies, failure to thrive, enzyme inducer, hemorrhage
ANTIMICROBIALS	
Ampicillin	All antimicrobials cross placenta ↓ Maternal urinary and plasma estriol levels
Chloramphenicol	Crosses placenta with no reported effect; interferes with biotransformation of tolbutamide, phenytoin, biohydroxycoumarin (i.e., hypoglycemia may occur if used in combination)
Chloroquine	Death, deafness, retinal hemorrhage
Erythromycin	Possible hepatic injury
Nitrofurantoin	Megaloblastic anemia, G6PD deficiency
Novobiocin	Hyperbilirubinemia

MATERNAL MEDICATION	REPORTED EFFECTS ON FETUS OR NEONATE
Streptomycin	Therapeutic levels reached, nerve deafness
Sulfonamides	Icterus, hemolytic anemia, kernicterus, growth retardation (?), thrombocytopenia
Tetracycline	Placental transfer after 4 months' gestation; enamel hypoplasia, delay in bone growth, congenital cataract (?)
ANTITUBERCULOSIS	
Isoniazid	Toxic blood level in fetus; no reported effect; mother should be on pyridoxine supplement
Pyridoxine	See vitamins
CANCER CHEMO-THERAPEUTIC AGENTS	
Aminopterin	Abortion, congenital anomalies (first trimester); combination of drugs detrimental to
6-Mercaptopurine	fetus; skeletal and cranial malformations, hydrocephalus; questionable long-term
Methotrexate	effects such as slow somatic growth; ovarian agenesis; ↓ immune mechanisms
CARDIOVASCULAR AGENTS	
Digitoxin	Placental transfer, no reported effect

Continued

Maternal Medication	Reported Effects on Fetus or Neonate
Propranolol	Indirect effect of delay in cervical dilatation
CHOLINESTERASE INHIBITORS	Myasthenia-like symptoms for 1 week; muscle weakness in 10% to 20% of infants
Cigarette smoking	Effect equal to number of cigarettes smoked; ↑ incidence of stillbirth; low-birth-weight; effect on later somatic growth and mental development (?); reduction in O_2 transport to fetus
DIURETICS	
Ammonium chloride	Maternal and fetal acidosis; thrombocytopenia, hemorrhage,
Thiazide	hypoelectrolytemia, convulsions, respiratory distress, death, hemolysis
DRUGS OF ABUSE (USUALLY MULTIPLE DRUGS CONSUMED)	
Alcohol	Blood level equal to mother's; convulsions, withdrawal syndrome, hyperactivity, crying, irritability, poor sucking reflex, low-birth-weight; cleft palate, ophthalmic malformation, malformation of extremities and heart; poor mental performance, microencephaly, small for dates, growth deficiency

Maternal Medication	Reported Effects on Fetus or Neonate
Barbiturates	Withdrawal symptoms, convulsions, onset immediately after birth or at 2 weeks of age
Cocaine	Abruptio placentae, preterm labor
"Ice"-methamphetamine	Preterm labor, IUGR, abnormal sleep patterns, poor feeding, tremors, hypertonia
LSD (lysergic acid diethylamide)	Chromosome breakage, limb and skeletal anomalies
Narcotics	Small for dates, 4% to 10% mortality, habituation, withdrawal symptoms,
Heroin	convulsions, sudden infant death syndrome (SIDS), indirect effect of maternal
Methadone	complications (i.e., infection, hepatitis, STD), permanent effect on somatic growth (?)
HORMONES	
Androgens	Labioscrotal fusion before week 12; after 12 weeks, phallic enlargement; other
Estrogens	anomalies (?); ↑ bilirubin (?), vaginal cancer; cleft lip and palate, CHD;
Progestins	tracheoesophageal fistula and atresia; cancer of prostate, testes, and bladder
Corticosteroids	Adrenal insufficiency, cleft palate, small-for-dates infant
Ovulatory agents	Anencephaly (?), chromosomal abnormalities in abortus (?), multiple pregnancy

Continued

MATERNAL MEDICATION	REPORTED EFFECTS ON FETUS OR NEONATE
PSYCHOTROPIC DRUGS	
Diazepam (Valium)	High fetal levels; hypotonia, poor sucking reflex, hypothermia; low APGAR score; ↑ resuscitation, ↑ assisted births; dose related
Lithium carbonate	Neonatal serum levels reach adult toxic range; lethargy, cyanosis for 10 days; teratogenic—dose related
RADIATION	Microencephaly, mental retardation, many unknown effects; nondisjunction of chromosomes
SEDATIVES	
Barbiturates	Apnea, depression, depressed electroencephalogram (EEG), poor sucking reflex, slow weight gain; concentration of drug in brain; enzyme inducer, lower bilirubin level
Bromides	Growth failure, lethargy, dilated pupils, dermatitis, hypotonia; effect on mental development(?)
Magnesium sulfate	Neonatal blood level does not correlate with clinical condition; respiratory depression, hypotonia, convulsions, death; exchange transfusion may be required
Paraldehyde	Apnea, depression

Maternal Medication	Reported Effects on Fetus or Neonate
Thalidomide	Administered between days 34 and 50 of gestation causes phocomelia, malformation of cord, angiomas of face, CHD, intestinal stenosis, eye defects, absence of appendix
TOXINS	
Carbon monoxide	Stillbirth, brain damage equal to anoxia
Heavy metals	
Arsenic	Concentrated in brain
Lead	Abortion, growth retardation, congenital anomalies, sterility
Mercury	Cerebral palsy, mental retardation, convulsions, involuntary movements, defective vision; mother asymptomatic
Naphthalene	Hemolysis
VITAMINS	
A and D	Congenital anomalies
K (water-soluble analogs)	Icterus, anemia, kernicterus
Pyridoxine	Withdrawal seizures

Appendix 8

Relationship of Drugs to Breast Milk and Effect on Infant

The drugs listed in this appendix have been categorized by their major use. The ratings given are those published by the American Academy of Pediatrics Committee on Drugs (AAP). These ratings label drugs that transfer into human milk. Drugs without a rating were not included in the AAP list. The ratings are described as:

1. Drugs that are contraindicated during breastfeeding
2. Drugs of abuse that are contraindicated during breastfeeding
3. Radioactive compounds that require temporary cessation of breastfeeding
4. Drugs with unknown effects on breastfeeding, but may be of concern
5. Drugs that have been associated with significant effects on some nursing infants and should be given to breastfeeding mothers with caution
6. Maternal medication usually compatible with breastfeeding
7. Food and environmental agents: effect on breastfeeding

DRUG	EXCRETED IN MILK	% ADULT DOSE IN MILK	AAP RATING	COMMENTS
ANALGESICS AND ANTIINFLAMMATORY DRUGS (NONNARCOTIC)				
Acetaminophen (Datril, Tylenol)	Yes	0.04 to 1.85	6	Detoxified in liver. Avoid in immediate postbirth period; otherwise no problems with therapeutic dose.
Aspirin (Bayer, Anacin, Bufferin, Excedrin, etc.)	Yes	10.55 ± 10.45	6	Long history of experience shows complications rare. Can cause interference with platelet aggregation and diminished factor XII (Hageman factor) at birth. When mother requires high, continuing level of medication for arthritis, aspirin is drug of choice. Observe infant for bruisability. Platelet aggregation can be evaluated. Salicylism only seen in maternal overdosing. Mother should increase vitamin C and vitamin K intake.

Continued

From Bobak IM, Lowdermilk DL, Jensen MD: *Maternity nursing*, ed 4, St Louis, 1995, Mosby.

Drug	Excreted in Milk	% Adult Dose in Milk	AAP Rating	Comments
ANALGESICS AND ANTIINFLAMMATORY DRUGS—CONT'D				
Ibuprofen (Advil, Nuprin, Motrin, etc.)	Yes	<0.8	6	No apparent effects in therapeutic doses.
Indomethacin (Indocin)	Yes	0.11 to 0.98	6	Convulsions in breastfed neonate (case report). Used to close patent ductus arteriosus. Insufficient data as to effect on other vessels. May be nephrotoxic.
Mefenamic acid (Ponstel)	Yes	0.036 to 0.8	6	No apparent effect on infant at therapeutic doses; infant able to excrete via urine.
Naproxen (Naproxyn, Anaprox, Naprosyn, Aleve)	Yes	1.1		Less toxic in adults than some other organic derivatives.
Propoxyphene (Darvon)	Yes	Trace amounts	6	Only symptoms detectable would be failure to feed and drowsiness. On daily, around-the-clock dosage, infant could consume 1 mg/day.

Drug	Excreted in Milk	% Adult Dose in Milk	AAP Rating	Comments
ANTIINFECTIVES (MAY CHANGE INTESTINAL FLORA OF INFANT AND SENSITIZE FOR LATER ALLERGIC REACTION)				
Acyclovir (Zovirax)	Yes	5.6 + 4.4	6	Minimal absorption through maternal skin.
Ampicillin (Polycillin, Amcill, Omnipen, Penbritin)	Yes	0.05 to 0.04		Sensitivity resulting from repeated exposure; diarrhea or secondary candidiasis.
Carbenicillin (Pyopen, Geopen)	Yes	0.001		Levels not significant. Drug is given to neonate. Not well absorbed from gastrointestinal tract.
Cefazolin (Ancef, Kefzol)	Yes	0.075	6	Probably not significant. Detected in milk if given IV.
Cephalexin (Keflex)	Yes	0.86 ± 0.35		Completely gone by 8 hours; absorption less in first few months.

Continued

DRUG	EXCRETED IN MILK	% ADULT DOSE IN MILK	AAP RATING	COMMENTS
ANTIINFECTIVES—CONT'D				
Cephalothin (Keflin)	Yes	0.4		Negligible.
Chloramphenicol (Chloromycetin)	Yes	1.6	4	Gray syndrome. Infant does not excrete drug well, and small amounts may accumulate. Contraindicated. May be tolerated in older infant with mature glycuronide system.
Colistin (Colymycin)	Yes	0.07		Not absorbed orally.
Demeclocycline (Declomycin)	Yes	Trace		Not significant in therapeutic doses. Can be given to infants. Drug remains in milk 3 days after dose.
Erythromycin (Ilosone, E-Mycin, Erythrocin)	Yes	0.1 to 2.1	6	Higher concentrations have been reported in milk than in plasma. Should not be given under 1 month of age because of risk of jaundice. Dose in milk higher when given IV to mother.
Gentamicin	Yes	Trace		Not absorbed from gastrointestinal tract, may change gut flora. Drug is given to newborns directly.
Isoniazid (Nydrazid)	Yes	2.3		Infant at risk for toxicity, but need for breast milk may outweigh risk.

Drug	Excreted in Milk	% Adult Dose in Milk	AAP Rating	Comments
Kanamycin (Kantrex)	Yes	0.95	6	Infant absorbs little from gastrointestinal tract. Infants can be given drug.
Metronidazole (Flagyl)	Yes	0.13 to 36	4	Caution should be exercised because of its high milk concentrations. Contraindicated when infant under 6 months; may cause neurologic disorders and blood dyscrasia. AAP says to discard milk for 12 hours if mother takes 2 g dose.
Nitrofurantoin (Furadantin, Macrodantin)	Yes	0.6	6	Not significant in therapeutic doses to affect child except in G6PD deficiency.
Novobiocin (Albamycin, Cathomycin)	Yes	0.15		Infant can be given drug directly.
Nystatin (Mycostatin)	No	Not absorbed orally		Can be given to infant directly.
Oxacillin (Prostaphilin)	No	Trace		Can be given to infant directly.

Continued

DRUG	EXCRETED IN MILK	% ADULT DOSE IN MILK	AAP RATING	COMMENTS
ANTIINFECTIVES—CONT'D				
Penicillin G, benzathine (Bicillin)	Yes	0.8		Clinical need should supersede possible allergic responses.
Penicillin G, potassium	Yes	0.8		Infant can be given penicillin directly. Parents should be told to inform physician that infant has been exposed to penicillin because of potential sensitivity.
Streptomycin	Yes	0.5	6	Not to be given more than 2 weeks. Ototoxic and nephrotoxic with long use. Is given to infants directly.
Sulfisoxazole (Gantrisin)	Yes	0.45	6	To be avoided during first month after birth; may cause kernicterus.
Tetracycline HCl (Achromycin, Panmycin, Sumycin)	Yes	0.3 to 4.8	6	Not enough to treat an infection in an infant. May cause discoloration of the teeth in the infant; the antibiotic, however, may be largely bound to the milk calcium. Do not give longer than 10 days or repeatedly.

DRUG	EXCRETED IN MILK	% ADULT DOSE IN MILK	AAP RATING	COMMENTS
ANTICOAGULANTS				
Coumarin derivatives	Yes	0.5	6	Monitor prothrombin time. Give vitamin K to infant. Discontinue if surgery or trauma occurs. Drug of choice if mother to continue breastfeeding. May cause bleeding.
Dicumarol (bishy-droxycoumarin) Warfarin (Panwarfin)				
Heparin	No			Heparin ineffective orally.
ANTICONVULSANTS AND SEDATIVES (BAR-BITURATES MAY PASS INTO MILK BUT DO NOT SEDATE INFANT)				
Magnesium sulfate	Yes	0.5	6	May produce sedation in infant.
Pentobarbital (Nembutal)	Yes	Traces		Depends on liver for detoxification so may accumulate in first week of life until infant is able to detoxify. No problem for older infant in usual doses.

Continued

Drug	Excreted in Milk	% Adult Dose in Milk	AAP Rating	Comments
ANTICONVULSANTS —CONT'D				
Phenobarbital (Luminal)	Yes	1.5	5	Sleepiness and decreased sucking possible. On usual analeptic doses infants alert and feed well. On hypnotic doses infants depressed and difficult to rouse.
Phenytoin (Dilantin)	Yes	1.4 to 7.2	6	No problem if mother's dose is in therapeutic range.
Sodium bromide (Bromo-Seltzer and across-the-counter sleeping aids)	Yes		6.7	Drowsy, decreased crying, rash, decreased feeding. No longer available in the United States.
ANTIHISTAMINES (MAY SUPPRESS LACTATION; ADMINISTER AFTER NURSING; ALL PASS INTO BREAST MILK)				

DRUG	EXCRETED IN MILK	% ADULT DOSE IN MILK	AAP RATING	COMMENTS
Brompheniramine (Dimetane)	Yes	Unknown		Drugs used in neonates. May cause sedation, decreased feeding, or may produce stimulation and tachycardia. Should avoid long-acting preparations, which may accumulate in infant.
Diphenhydramine (Benadryl)	Yes	Unknown		When combined with decongestants, may cause decrease in milk.
Promethazine (Phenergan)	Yes	Unknown	6	Passage into breast is expected; increases serum prolactin levels.
AUTONOMIC DRUGS				
Atropine sulfate*	Yes	Traces	6	Hyperthermia, atropine toxicity, infants especially sensitive; also inhibits lactation. Infant dose 0.01 mg/kg.
Ergotamine	Yes	Unknown	1	May inhibit lactation.
Neostigmine	No			No known harm to infant.

*An ingredient in many prescription and nonprescription drugs.

Continued

DRUG	EXCRETED IN MILK	% ADULT DOSE IN MILK	AAP RATING	COMMENTS
AUTONOMIC DRUGS—CONT'D				
Propantheline bromide (Pro-Banthine)	No	Uncontrolled data indicate no measurable levels.	1	Drug rapidly metabolized in maternal system to inactive metabolite. Mother should avoid long-acting preparations, however.
Scopolamine (Hyoscine)	Yes	Traces	6	Usually given as single dose and of no problem to neonate. No data on repeated doses.
CARDIOVASCULAR DRUGS				
Diazoxide (Hyperstat)				Arteriolar dilators and antihypertensive, only given IV, not active orally.
Digoxin	Yes	0.07 to 14	6	Not detected in infant's plasma.
Hydralazine (Apresoline)	Yes	0.8	6	Jaundice, thrombocytopenia, electrolyte disturbances possible.
Methyldopa (Aldomet)	Yes	0.02 to 0.09		Galactorrhea. No specific data except as affects mother's milk production.

DRUG	EXCRETED IN MILK	% ADULT DOSE IN MILK	AAP RATING	COMMENTS
Propranolol (Inderal)	Yes	Traces		Insignificant amount. Infants reported had no symptoms noted. Should watch for hypoglycemia and/or "β-blocking" effects.
Quinidine	Yes	4.1	6	Arrhythmia may occur.
CATHARTICS				
Cascara	Yes	Low	6	Caused colic and diarrhea in infant.
Milk of Magnesia	No	None	6	No effect.
Mineral oil	No	None	6	No effect.
Phenolphthalein	Unknown	Unknown	6	Reported to cause symptoms in some.
Rhubarb	Unknown	None	6	None in syrup form. Fresh rhubarb may give symptoms of colic and diarrhea.
Saline cathartics	No	None	6	No effect.
Senna	No	None	6	None.
Stool softeners and bulk-forming laxatives	No	None	6	No effect.

Continued

Drug	Excreted in Milk	% Adult Dose in Milk	AAP Rating	Comments
CATHARTICS—CONT'D				
Suppositories (for constipation)	No	None		Not absorbed.
DIURETICS				
Furosemide (sulfamylan-thranilic acid) (Lasix)	Possible	Not found in all samples	6	Drug is given to children under medical management.
Spironolactone (Aldactone)	Yes	Canrenone, a metabolite, appears	6	Acts as antagonist of aldosterone; causes sodium excretion and potassium retention. The metabolite apparently has some activity.
Thiazides (Diuril, Enduron, Esidrix, Hydrodiuril, Oretic, Thiuretic tablets)	Yes	0.25 to 0.43	6	Risk of dehydration and electrolyte imbalance, especially sodium loss, which would require monitoring. Watching weight and wet diapers and taking an occasional specific gravity reading of urine and serum sodium wold indicate status of infant. Risk, however, is extremely low. May suppress lactation because of dehydration in mother.

Drug	Excreted in Milk	% Adult Dose in Milk	AAP Rating	Comments
ENVIRONMENTAL AGENTS				
Benzene hexachloride (BHC)	Yes	Varies by location	7	Not a reason to wean from breast. No need to test milk unless inordinate exposure.
Dichlorodiphenyl trichlorethane (DDT or DDE)	Yes	Varies by location	7	Not a reason to wean from breast. No need to test milk unless inordinate exposure.
Methyl mercury	Yes	Varies by location	7	Infant blood level 600 ng/ml in heavy exposure. Only in excessive exposure is testing and/or weaning necessary.
Polybrominated biphenyl (PBB)	Yes	Varies by location	7	If mother at high risk from the environment or the diet, milk sample should be measured. If level in milk is high, then breastfeeding should be discontinued. Those at risk are workers who handle PBB/PCB and individuals who eat game fish from contaminated waters. Crash diets mobilize fats and should be avoided, especially if PBB or PCB is present.
Polychlorinated biphenyl (PCB)	Yes	Varies by location	7	

Continued

Drug	Excreted in Milk	% Adult Dose in Milk	AAP Rating	Comments
HEAVY METALS				
Arsenic	Yes	Can be measured for given woman.		Can accumulate. Check infant's blood level if there is reason to suspect exposure.
Fluorine	Yes	0.19		Monitor for excessive dose. Depends on level in water supply.
Iron	Yes			
Lead	Unknown			Nursing contraindicated if maternal serum 40 µg; conflicting reports, breast milk not always cause of lead poisoning in breastfed infant.
Mercury	Yes		7	Hazardous to infant.
HORMONES AND CONTRACEPTIVES				
Chlorotrianisene (Tace)	Yes			Has estrogenic effect although does not change consistency of milk. May have feminizing effect on infant. May suppress lactation.

DRUG	EXCRETED IN MILK	% ADULT DOSE IN MILK	AAP RATING	COMMENTS
Contraceptives (oral) Ethinyl estradiol, Mestranol, 19-Nortestosterone, Norethindrone (Norlutin)	Yes	0.16 ± 0.14	6	May diminish milk supply. May decrease vitamins, protein, and fat in milk. Most significant concern is long-range impact of hormone on young infant, which is not certain. Reports of feminization of infant.
Corticotropin	Yes	1.1	6	May decrease quantity and quality of milk.
Cortisone	Yes	Significant amounts		May affect infant in therapeutic doses.
Epinephrine (Adrenalin)	Yes			Destroyed in gastrointestinal tract of infant.
Estrogen	Yes	0.1	6	Risks as with oral contraceptives. May alter quality and quantity of milk.
Insulin	No			Destroyed in intestinal tract.
Medroxyprogesterone acetate (Provera)	Yes	0.86 to 5	6	6-month injection may affect milk supply; 3-month injection should not decrease supply.

Continued

Drug	Excreted in Milk	% Adult Dose in Milk	AAP Rating	Comments
HORMONES AND CONTRACEPTIVES—CONT'D				
Prednisone	Yes	0.06 to 3.6	6	Minimum amount not likely to cause effect on infant in short course.
Tolbutamide (Orinase)	Yes	18	6	Watch for jaundice.
NARCOTICS				
Cocaine	Yes	Significant levels in milk	1,2	No metabolites or drug found in milk after 36 hours or in infant's urine after 60 hours.
Codeine	Yes	5 ± 2	6	No effect in therapeutic level and transient usage. Can accumulate. Individual variation. Watch for neonatal depression.
Heroin	Yes		2	Chinese metabolize drug less than Caucasians.
Marijuana (Cannabis)	Yes		2	Shown in laboratory animals to produce structural changes in nursling's brain cells; impairs DNA and RNA formation. Infant at risk of inhaling smoke during feeding or when held by person who is smoking.

DRUG	EXCRETED IN MILK	% ADULT DOSE IN MILK	AAP RATING	COMMENTS
Meperidine (Demerol)	Yes	Trace		Trace amounts may accumulate if drug taken around the clock when infant is neonate. Watch for drowsiness and poor feeding.
Methadone	Yes	2.2	6	When dosage not excessive, infant can be breastfed if monitored for evidence of depression and failure to thrive. Suggest mother get daily dose after evening feeding and supplement formula at next feeding.
Morphine	Yes	0.8 to 1.2	6	Single doses have minimum effect. Potential for accumulation. May be addicting to neonate. Breastfeeding no longer considered appropriate means of weaning infant of an addict.
Percodan (oxycodone [derived from opiate thebaine] aspirin, phenacetin, caffeine)	Yes	Unknown		Consider for its component parts. In neonatal period sleepiness and failure to feed, which increase maternal engorgement and neonatal weight loss, have been observed, probably caused by oxycodone.

Continued

Drug	Excreted in Milk	% Adult Dose in Milk	AAP Rating	Comments
PSYCHOTROPIC AND MOOD-CHANGING DRUGS				
Alcohol (ethanol)	Yes	1 to 19.5	6	Milk may smell like alcohol. Ethanol in doses of 1 to 2 g/kg to mother causes depression of milk-ejection reflex (dose dependent). No acetaldehyde found as infant cannot metabolize ethanol.
Amphetamine	Yes	6.1 ± 0.1	2	Has caused stimulation in infants with jitteriness, irritability, sleeplessness. Long-acting preparations cumulative.
Benzodiazepines* Chlordiazepoxide (Librium)	Yes			Not sufficient to affect infant first week when glucuronyl system needed for detoxification. May accumulate. May cause jaundice. Older infant, no apparent problem.
Diazepam (Valium)	Yes	2 to 4.7	4	Detoxified in glucuronyl system. In first weeks of life may contribute to jaundice. Metabolite active.

*Alcohol enhances the effects of these drugs.

Drug	Excreted in Milk	% Adult Dose in Milk	AAP Rating	Comments
				Effect on infant: hypoventilation, drowsiness, lethargy, and weight loss. Single doses over 10 mg contraindicated during breastfeeding. Accumulation in infant possible.
Haloperidol (Haldol)	Yes	0.15 to 2	4	A butyrophenone antidepressant: animal studies in nurslings show behavior abnormalities.
Lithium carbonate (Eskalith, Lithane, Lithonate)	Yes	1.8		Measurable lithium in infant's serum. Infant kidney can clear lithium; however, lithium inhibits adenosine 3':5'-cyclic monophosphate, significant for brain growth. Also affects amine metabolism. Report of cyanosis and poor muscle tone and ECG changes in nursing infant.
Meprobamate (Miltown, Equanil)	Yes	2 to 4 times maternal plasma level		If therapy continued, infant should be followed closely.
Phencyclidine (PCP)	Yes		1	Animal studies show PCP in milk even after drug has been discontinued for 40 days.

Continued

Drug	Excreted in Milk	% Adult Dose in Milk	AAP Rating	Comments
PSYCHOTROPIC AND MOOD-CHANGING DRUGS—CONT'D				
Phenothiazines Chlorpromazine (Thorazine)	Yes	0.07 to 0.2		Drowsiness and lethargy in infants.
Thioridazine (Mellaril)	Yes	No information		Thioridazine is less potent in general than other phenothiazines. Probably safe.
Trifluoperazine (Stelazine)	Yes	Minimum		
Tricyclic antidepressants Amitriptyline (Elavil)	Yes	0.8 ± 0.2	4	Apparently no accumulation. No infants under observation have shown symptoms.
Desipramine (Norpramin, Pertofrane)		1	4	Watch for depression or failure to feed. Increase maternal prolactin secretion.

Drug	Excreted in Milk	% Adult Dose in Milk	AAP Rating	Comments
Imipramine (Tofranil)	Yes	0.1	4	
STIMULANTS				
Caffeine	Yes	0.66 to 10	6	Accumulates when intake moderate and continual. Causes jitteriness, wakefulness, and irritability. Caffeine present in many hot and cold drinks. Consider if infant very wakeful.
Theobromine	Yes	20	7	No adverse symptoms observed in the infants. Chocolate the most common cause of exposure.
Theophylline	Yes	<1 to 15	6	Irritability, fretfulness.
THYROID AND ANTITHYROID MEDICATIONS				
Thiouracil	Yes	0.3 to 2.6	6	Get baseline levels of T3, T4, and TSH before and 6 weeks after mother starts medication.

Continued

DRUG	EXCRETED IN MILK	% ADULT DOSE IN MILK	AAP RATING	COMMENTS
THYROID AND ANTITHYROID MEDICATIONS—CONT'D				
Thyroid and thyroxine	Yes	0.3 to 2.6	6	Does not produce adverse symptoms on long-range follow-up. Noted to improve milk supply of mothers with hypothyroidism. No contraindications.
MISCELLANEOUS				
Diphtheria-pertussis-tetanus (DPT)	Yes	Minimum		Does not interfere with immunization schedule.
Methotrexate	Yes	0.93	1	Antimetabolite. Infant would receive 0.26 µg/dl, which researchers consider nontoxic for infant.
Nicotine	Yes		2	Decreases milk production. Smoking may interfere with let-down reflex if smoking started before onset of a feeding. Smoke exposure may be a concern.

Drug	Excreted in Milk	% Adult Dose in Milk	AAP Rating	Comments
Poliovirus vaccine	No			Live vaccine taken orally. Not necessary to withhold nursing 30 minutes before and after dose. Provide booster after infant no longer nursing.
Rh antibodies	Yes			Destroyed in gastrointestinal tract; not effective orally.
Rubella virus vaccine	Yes	Minimum		Will not confer passive immunity. Mother should not be given vaccine when at risk for pregnancy.
Tuberculin test	No			Tuberculin-sensitive mothers can adaptively immunize their infants through breast milk, and that immunity may last several years.
Chest x-ray				No effect.

BIBLIOGRAPHY

Creasy R, Resnick F, eds: *Maternal-fetal medicine: principles and practice,* Philadelphia, 1984, WB Saunders.

Cunningham FG et al: *Williams obstetrics,* ed 19, Norwalk, 1993, Appleton & Lange.

Eronen M et al: The effects of indomethacin and a *B*-sympathomimetic agent on the fetal ductus arteriosus during treatment of premature labor: a randomized double-blind study, *Am J Obstet Gynecol* 164:141-146, 1991.

Fischbach F: *A manual of laboratory diagnostic tests,* ed 2, Philadelphia, 1984, Lippincott.

Health Care Resources: *High-risk perinatal home care manual,* St Louis, 1997, Mosby.

Physician's desk reference, New York, 1995, Medical Economics Company.

Ridgway L et al: A prospective randomized comparison of oral terbutaline and magnesium oxide for the maintenance of tocolysis, *Am J Obstet Gynecol* 163:879-882, 1990.

Sabbagha RE: Dept. of Obstetrics & Gynecology, Northwestern University.

Sibai BM: Management of preeclampsia, *Clin Perinatol Hypertens Pregnancy* 18:793-808, 1991.

I N D E X